Socioeconomic Characteristics of Medical Practice 1983

Roger A. Reynolds
Jonathan B. Abram
Editors

Center for Health Policy Research

The information contained in this volume is from the AMA
Socioeconomic Monitoring System. The AMA Center for Health
Policy Research directs the Socioeconomic Monitoring System
in cooperation with the AMA Division of Survey and Data
Resources.

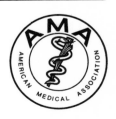

21145

Additional copies of this book
may be purchased from:
Order Department OP 165
American Medical Association
P.O. Box 10946
Chicago, Illinois 60610

KDB:83-544:5M:9/83

ISBN 0-89970-165-5

SOCIOECONOMIC CHARACTERISTICS OF MEDICAL PRACTICE

Table of Contents

LIST OF TABLES

**Patient Care Activities: Psychiatry, Radiology, Anesthesiology,
and Pathology**

Waiting Time

Hospital Utilization

Fees

Professional Expenses

Net Income

FOREWORD

A rapidly changing medical practice environment is confronting physicians, policymakers and the public with changing choices. The ability to make well-informed decisions in response to these changes requires the availability of detailed and timely information on socioeconomic aspects of medicine. <u>Socioeconomic Characteristics of Medical Practice</u> (or "Gray Book") is meant to meet, in part, this need.

Although this is the first edition of the Gray Book, the American Medical Association has been collecting and disseminating information on the socioeconomic characteristics of medicine since 1966. Until 1980, this information was collected through annual mail surveys of physicians known as the Periodic Survey of Physicians and published in the <u>Profile of Medical Practice</u> series.

The Socioeconomic Monitoring System (SMS), introduced in late 1981, replaced the methodology of the Periodic Surveys with quarterly telephone surveys of physicians. This change was made to respond to the need for more frequent and timely information. A detailed overview of SMS is provided in the article by Sharon R. Henderson and Mary Lou S. White at the beginning of this volume. This is followed by reprints of selected recent issues of the <u>SMS Report</u> — a frequently published newsletter that facilitates rapid dissemination of SMS results -- on topics of current health policy interest.

The main body of the Gray Book is devoted to providing detailed tabulations of trends and variations in a range of characteristics of physician's practices including aspects of practice activities, fees, income and expenses. This volume also contains a comprehensive summary of information on practice characteristics in 1982 based on SMS surveys conducted throughout the past year.

A program of the magnitude of SMS has required a major commitment from many individuals. Although I am grateful to all who have contributed to various aspects of SMS, it is impossible to mention each individually. However, I would particularly like to thank Norbert W. Budde, Ph.D., Director of the Division of Survey and Data Resources, whose division has cooperated with the Center for Health Policy Research in many of the activities relating to SMS.

Lynn E. Jensen, Ph.D.
Director
Center for Health Policy Research

INTRODUCTION

Socioeconomic Characteristics of Medical Practice (the Gray Book) is designed as an annual reference volume on data collected by the AMA Socioeconomic Monitoring System (SMS). The Gray Book maintains the tradition of the AMA, established in past by Profile of Medical Practice series, as a primary source of baseline data on socioeconomic aspects of medicine.

This volume is primarily devoted to providing detailed information on medical practice characteristics in 1982 based on information data collected by SMS surveys. In addition, trends are shown for characteristics for which similar data was collected in the past by AMA Periodic Survey of Physicians (PSPs). In order to maintain continuity with the past, every effort has been made to ensure that data reported in the Gray Book from the PSPs is consistent with information in the Profile of Medical Practice 1981.

We caution users of the trend data to carefully note differences between the methodology used in collecting data in the PSPs and SMS, since these differences may indicate apparent rather than real changes in characteristics over time. Differences in the methodology of SMS from the PSPs are discussed by Sharon R. Henderson and Mary Lou S. White in their article on the "Design and Methodology of the AMA Socioeconomic Monitoring System" and further elaborated in the appendixes.

We have benefited from the guidance and assistance of many individuals in the planning and preparation of this first edition of the Gray Book. We are particularly grateful to Lynn E. Jensen and Jack L. Werner, Director and Assistant Director, respectively, of the Center for Health Policy Research, who provided comments and advice at all stages of the development of this volume and to Don Pieniazek for his expert secretarial assistance.

Roger A. Reynolds
Jonathan B. Abram

August, 1983

THE DESIGN AND METHODOLOGY OF THE AMA
SOCIOECONOMIC MONITORING SYSTEM

by Sharon R. Henderson and Mary Lou S. White*

The Socioeconomic Monitoring System (SMS) was developed in 1981 in response to the need of physicians and policymakers for more timely and frequent socioeconomic information on the practice of medicine than has been available in the past. This new survey program represents an outgrowth of over 15 years of AMA experience in monitoring socioeconomic aspects of medical practice. Like its predecessor, the Periodic Survey of Physicians (PSP), SMS was designed to provide information on a range of baseline characteristics of medical practice, including physicians' earnings, expenses, work patterns and fees.

SMS, however, offers several improvements over PSP:

- Frequency: Compared with the annual basis on which PSP data were collected, SMS surveys are conducted four times each year, once each quarter.

- Timeliness of Results: Telephone interviews are used by SMS in contrast to the PSP mail questionnaire methodology in order to collect information and disseminate results more rapidly.

- Expanded Population Coverage: In recognition of their growing importance in the physician population, hospital-associated physicians are included in the population from which SMS samples are drawn, as well as the office-based physician population on which PSP was traditionally based.

- Responsiveness to Policy Concerns: A portion of each SMS survey is devoted to collecting information regarding to current policy issues relating to the practice of medicine.

The purpose of this paper is to provide a detailed description of the current SMS program design. The first section provides an overview of program characteristics. This is followed by discussions of the SMS survey sample design, questionnaire content, field procedures and aspects of the reporting SMS results.

---

*Sharon R. Henderson is Director, Office of Corporate Planning and Analysis and Mary Lou S. White is Assistant Director of the Department of Survey Design and Analysis, Division of Survey and Data Resources, American Medical Association.

OVERVIEW OF SMS PROGRAM CHARACTERISTICS

The four SMS surveys conducted each year include an annual core survey and three supplemental quarterly surveys. The annual and quarterly surveys differ in the range of information collected, sample size and the level of detail for which results are reported. The purpose of the annual core survey is to provide current data on a full range of economic and practice characteristics each year. The quarterly surveys focus on a more limited range of characteristics — those for which changes occur rapidly and those for which information is needed on a more frequent basis. The quarterly surveys are also used to obtain information on topics of current policy concern. The average core survey interview lasts 25 minutes, while quarterly surveys average 16 minutes in length.

The annual core survey obtains data from approximately 4,000 physicians, while the quarterly surveys obtain data from approximately 1,200 physicians each. The sample size is the primary determinant of the level of disaggregation at which results can be reliably reported. Results are disaggregated into a larger number of specialties and geographical areas for the core survey than for individual quarterly surveys.

The annual core survey is fielded in the second calendar quarter of each year, beginning in early April. The timing of the beginning of the core survey is designed to coincide with the income tax return filing deadline in order to improve the reliability of information that can be obtained on physician earnings and practice expenses for the previous year. The quarterly surveys begin during the first weeks in January, July and October. The field periods for the core and supplemental quarterly surveys are respectively eight and six weeks.

The first SMS survey was conducted in the fourth quarter of 1981. The first full SMS program year, including four surveys, was completed in 1982.

SAMPLE DESIGN

The SMS surveys are designed to provide representative information on the population of all non-federal physicians, excluding residents, who spend the greatest proportion of their time in patient care activities. Thus, SMS surveys provide broader coverage of the physician population than the AMA's previous socioeconomic surveys, which were limited to office-based physicians. This difference in population coverage should be kept in mind when contrasting information on physicians' practices from SMS surveys with information for years prior to 1981 from the PSPs.

Samples for SMS surveys are selected from the AMA Physician Masterfile. The Masterfile contains current and historical information on every Doctor of Medicine in the United States, including both members and non-members of the AMA. Graduates of U.S. medical schools who are temporarily practicing overseas, and graduates of foreign medical schools who live in the U.S. are also included on the file.

Data included on the Masterfile are obtained only from primary sources including many organizations and institutions. The only information obtained directly from individual physicians concerns current professional activities and preferred mailing addresses. These data are obtained on a quadrennial basis from the entire U.S. physician population and on a monthly basis from those physicians with changes in address or professional status. These changes may be signalled by input from professional organizations, AMA mailings, or by physician correspondence.

The main categories of physicians excluded from the population used in selecting survey samples from the Masterfile are as follows:

- physicians whose major professional activity is medical teaching, administration, research or some other activity not involving direct patient care;

- residents;

- Doctors of Osteopathy;

- federally employed physicians;

- graduates of foreign medical schools who are only temporarily licensed to practice in the United States;

- physicians for whom no current address is available, and

- physicians who were sampled for PSP or SMS during the last three years.

Further exclusions are made after sample selection. These include:

- physicians who spend fewer than 20 hours per week in patient care or are federal physicians as determined screening questions at the beginning of each interview, and

- those who are unlocatable by mail or telephone after exhaustive tracking efforts are made.

The sample design utilized for all surveys is a stratified, random sample with systematic selection from the listing of eligible physicians on the AMA Physician Masterfile. The strata are defined by nine major specialty groupings and ten geographical regions of approximately equal size. Systematic selection within each stratum assures that each specialty group and region is proportionally represented in the sample. The strata definitions are shown in Table 1. Stratification is used in SMS to increase the precision of certain of the sample estimates and to facilitate the analysis of individual strata.

Table 1

SMS SURVEY SAMPLE STRATA

SPECIALTY STRATA*

1. General Practice, Family Practice

2. Allergy, Cardiovascular Diseases, Gastroenterology, Internal Medicine, Pulmonary Diseases

3. General Surgery, Neurosurgery, Ophthalmology, Orthopedic Surgery, Plastic Surgery, Colon and Rectal Surgery, Thoracic Surgery, Urology

4. Pediatrics, Pediatric Allergy, Pediatric Cardiology

5. Obstetrics and Gynecology

6. Radiology, Diagnostic Radiology, Therapeutic Radiology

7. Psychiatry, Child Psychiatry

8. Anesthesiology

9. Aerospace Medicine, Neurology, Occupational Medicine, Physical Medicine and Rehabilitation, General Preventive Medicine, Public Health, Dermatology, Pathology, Forensic Pathology, Other Specialty, Unspecified

STATE STRATA

1. Connecticut, Maine, Massachusetts, New Hampshire, Rhode Island, Vermont

2. New York

3. Delaware, New Jersey, Pennsylvania, West Virginia

4. District of Columbia, Georgia, Maryland, North Carolina, South Carolina, Virginia

5. Alabama, Florida, Kentucky, Mississippi, Tennessee

6. Arkansas, Louisiana, Missouri, Oklahoma, Texas

7. Indiana, Michigan, Ohio

8. Illinois, Iowa, Minnesota, Wisconsin

9. Alaska, Arizona, Colorado, Hawaii, Idaho, Kansas, Montana, Nevada, Nebraska, New Mexico, North Dakota, South Dakota, Oregon, Utah, Wyoming, Washington

10. California

---

*The AMA Physician Masterfile classification of specialties is used in the specialty strata listing.

In order to provide reliable estimates of short-term changes in certain indicators, SMS samples are designed to include a panel component. The panel consists of a portion of the sample from one SMS survey which is reinterviewed in a subsequent SMS survey. During 1982, the size and frequency of reinterviewing for the SMS panel component has varied in order to provide useful information in determining the most efficient design for future SMS surveys. In most SMS surveys, approximately 40 percent of the completed interviews were conducted as reinterviews with physicians who had been initially interviewed in the preceding quarter. In some SMS surveys, however, the panel component also included a portion of reinterviews with physicians who had been initially interviewed in the same quarter of the previous year.

QUESTIONNAIRE CONTENT

The SMS questionnaire consists of three distinct sections:

- <u>screening questions</u> to verify the physician's specialty and eligibility for the survey;

- <u>a main questionnaire</u> to collect information on practice, characteristics, hours worked, volume of services, fees for selected procedures, income and expenses; and

- <u>special topics questions</u> to provide information on emerging socioeconomic issues.

The screening and main questionnaire portion of the survey remain unchanged every quarter to provide the basis for estimating levels and changes in economic characteristics of medical practice. However, the core survey includes an expanded main questionnaire portion to provide additional information on practice characteristics and final information on annual income and expenses for the previous year. This expanded portion remains constant from one core survey to the next.

Questions for the main questionnaire were developed from a review of past surveys and through consultation with physicians, sources within the AMA and Mathematica Policy Research, Inc., an independent consulting firm that assisted in the development of the SMS program. Efforts were made to maintain consistency of questions with those from the PSPs from which trend information has been established over a period of years. However, modifications were made where it was deemed that the desired information would be more accurate if questions were changed. In addition, questions in the SMS surveys are designed so that physicians are asked only questions that are generally relevant to their specialty. This contrasts with the use of the same questionnaire for physicians in all specialties in the PSPs. A summary of the questionnaire used in the SMS surveys is included in Appendix A.

Special topics questions vary with each survey. The topics covered since the first SMS survey have included:

- Physician Financial Arrangements with Hospitals
- Ambulatory Surgery
- Medical Technology Diffusion
- Malpractice Claims Experience
- Physician/Hospital Relations
- Physician Responses to Competition

Special topics questions are formulated and reviewed by an AMA consultation committee whose members represent a broad range of activity areas. These questions are pretested prior to the survey fielding to evaluate the wording and ordering of questions and to determine the ability of respondents to provide the desired information.

FIELD PROCEDURES

The SMS data collection plan is designed to provide reliable information within a tight time schedule. The survey is completed primarily by telephone. Telephone administration significantly reduces the time required to produce survey results and increases the response rate. The surveys are administered by independent consulting firms contracted by the AMA. The fourth quarter 1981, first quarter 1982, and the second quarter 1983 surveys were conducted by Mathematica Policy Research, Inc. of Princeton, New Jersey. Surveys for the second quarter 1982 through the first quarter 1983 were conducted by Chilton Research Services of Radnor, Pennsylvania.

Field procedures developed for SMS surveys reflect a complex effort to minimize bias from nonresponse and accomodate the busy schedule of physicians through careful advance preparation and intensive follow-up efforts to complete interviews. The activities involved in this effort are described below.

Advance Letter

Two weeks prior to data collection, advance letters are sent to each physician selected to be interviewed or reinterviewed. The letters are basically the same for the two sample groups, but those addressed to the reinterview sample are thanked for their past cooperation. Each letter includes a brief description of the interview, the project sponsorship, identification of the survey contractor, information that the physician will be receiving a telephone call from an interviewer on the contractor's staff, and a pledge of data confidentiality. Each letter is printed on AMA letterhead and bears the signature of James H. Sammons, M.D., Executive Vice President of the American Medical Association. If a letter is returned due to an insufficient address, a search is initiated to obtain updated information so the physician may be sent another letter. Beginning with the third quarter 1983 survey, a questionnaire summary is being enclosed with each advance letter to enable physicians to better prepare for the survey.

Telephone Search

Approximately two weeks prior to data collection, the survey contractor is provided names and addresses of physicians selected from the AMA Physician Masterfile. At this point, telephone "look up" is attempted. Since inadequate coverage is a potential problem for telephone surveys, considerable effort is expended to locate sample physicians.

The basic sources used in the telephone look-up include directory assistance, state and county medical societies, state licensing boards and hospitals. If the survey contractor is unable to obtain a telephone listing for a physician from these sources, the AMA Division of Survey and Data Resources lends assistance by reverifying the physicians' data contained on the AMA Physician Masterfile, contacting state, county and specialty societies, initiating traces of physicians from former addresses appearing on the Masterfile and checking medical society directories.

Interviewer Training

Two days of study-specific training in adddition to general training are provided to each interviewer before working on SMS surveys. Training includes a detailed review of each question (including instruction on pronunciation of various medical terms), practice interviews, and a review of interviewing and administrative procedures. AMA staff actively participate in the training process either in person or via teleconferencing as insurance that all project specifications and instructions are clearly communicated, understood, and implemented.

During training, the contractor actively evaluates each potential interviewer for appropriate survey skills, such as reading ability, voice quality, grasp of the material and ability to develop rapport with physicians. The highest quality interviewers are then selected to work on the project.

Interview Process

Interviewing is conducted via a Computer Assisted Telephone Interviewing (CATI) process. This system produces a copy of the questionnaire on a computer screen. Responses to the questions are entered directly into the computer using this on-line system during the actual interview, eliminating any keypunching or separate data entry task. This reduces time schedules and maximizes quality by minimizing sources of error.

A minimum of a 60 percent response rate is required in order to regard an SMS survey as complete. Vigorous efforts are be made in order to achieve the cooperation of physicians and meet this standard because of the short field period of SMS surveys. These efforts include the following:

- Appointments for interviews are scheduled at the convenience of physicians at any time 13 hours a day from Monday through Saturday.

- A toll-free number allows physicians to complete the interview at their convenience.

- An optional mail questionnaire, tailored to each specialty and type of practice, is made available to physicians who indicate a preference for responding to the survey in writing rather than by telephone.

- Repeated callbacks (a minimum of four) to nonrespondents are made before abandoning efforts to interview the physician.

- Refusal conversion attempts are made by a select group of interviewers. A substantive number of physician decide to grant an interview at this stage.

The actual response rates achieved in SMS surveys through the 2nd quarter of 1983 are shown in Table 2. The results indicate the success SMS has had in meeting its minimum 60 percent response rate standard.

Quality Control

Each interviewer's work is monitored by the contractor's supervisory staff for both production and quality. AMA staff remotely monitor on-going surveys conducted by each interviewer to ensure that a high quality level is maintained throughout the survey. This involves actually listening to the interviews being conducted on a periodic basis. If indicated, the contractor is instructed to retrain interviewers or remove unacceptable interviewers from the SMS study.

AMA staff also monitor the SMS survey production. A detailed review is made of all sample dispositions, both pending and final, on a weekly basis. As this evaluation is conducted, the time schedule is evaluated and necessary recommendations are made to the contractor to ensure that the time schedule is met.

Confidentiality

Data are entered via the CATI system and are released only in aggregate form without any individual respondent identifying information.

REPORTING OF SMS RESULTS

Results obtained from SMS surveys are disseminated widely. The SMS Report, a newsletter, is published approximately eight times a year to provide rapid dissemination of survey results. In order to reach the physician community, results are also published periodically in AMNews. Dissemination of information pertinent to the public is handled by the AMA Department of Public Information. Socioeconomic Characteristics of Medical Practice, or the "Gray Book", is an annual volume designed to provide more detailed results of SMS surveys than can generally be provided through other media.

TABLE 2

Number of Completed Interviews and Response Rates in SMS Surveys, 4th Quarter 1981 to 2nd Quarter 1983

Survey	Number of Completed Interviews	Response Rate
4th Quarter 1981	1,329	60.5%
1st Quarter 1982	1,213	70.2
2nd Quarter 1982 (Core Survey)	3,817	60.3
3rd Quarter 1982	1,247	60.8
4th Quarter 1982	1,215	62.7
1st Quarter 1983	1,237	65.0
2nd Quarter 1983 (Core Survey)	3,951	61.8

Data from the SMS also serve as a basis for research on health policy issues. Analyses of such issues are disseminated through professional journals and conferences. This ensures that health policy analysts and researchers are apprised of important findings resulting from this program.

Results from SMS surveys are reported at differing levels of detail depending on the nature of the media and the degree of precision of the estimates of physician characteristics deemed appropriate for the report. A discussion of definitions and computation procedures employed in reporting SMS results is contained in Appendix B.

CONCLUSION

The Socioeconomic Monitoring System exemplifies a long-term commitment on the part of the American Medical Association to obtain valid and reliable socioeconomic information on the practice of medicine. The SMS Program complements AMA's other extensive data collection activities and represents an important step in the evolution of these activities to meet the challenges of the 1980's.

PHYSICIANS' FINANCIAL ARRANGEMENTS WITH HOSPITALS*

This report explores the changing nature of financial arrangements between physicians and hospitals, including:

- the percentage of physicians with a hospital financial arrangement;

- the impact of hospital contracts on physicians' incomes; and

- the type and frequency of these contracts.

The data are from AMA's Socioeconomic Monitoring System (SMS). The information is obtained from the first SMS telephone survey which was conducted in the fourth quarter of 1981. The sample of respondents consists of 1,329 nonfederal patient care physicians, excluding residents.

Physicians With Hospital Contracts

Approximately one-fourth or 78,600 of all nonfederal patient care physicians, excluding residents, have some financial arrangement with hospitals in 1981 (see Table 1). Including residents and federal physicians, who also have hospital arrangements, the total rises to approximately 156,000 physicians.

Among specialists, pathologists (78%) and radiologists (58%) are those most likely to have financial contracts with hospitals.

Physicians in the fields of obstetrics (10%), surgery (11%), and general/family practice (14%) are least likely to have some financial arrangement with hospitals.

It is important to note that physicians specializing in emergency medicine, who probably have the largest number of agreements with hospitals, are not separately identified in this sample. They are counted in the "Other Specialties" category in Table 1.

*Reprinted from SMS Report Volume 1, No. 2, February 1982.

Table 1

NONFEDERAL PATIENT CARE PHYSICIANS WITH FINANCIAL
CONTRACTS WITH HOSPITALS, BY SPECIALTY

Specialty	Total Physicians*	Percent With Financial Arrangements	Estimated Number with Arrangements
ALL PHYSICIANS	302,300	26%	78,600
Pathology	8,500	78	6,600
Radiology	15,800	58	9,200
Internal Medicine	58,900	36	21,200
Other Specialties	26,000	35	7,500
Psychiatry	22,400	32	7,200
Anesthesiology	13,100	27	3,500
Pediatrics	20,300	17	3,500
General/Family Practice	50,600	14	7,100
Surgery	66,000	11	7,300
Obstetrics/Gynecology	20,700	10	2,100

*Source: Bidese, C. and D. Danais, Physician Characteristics and Distribu-
tion in the U. S. - 1981, Division of Survey and Data Resources,
American Medical Association, Chicago, Illinois.

Physicians' Incomes and Hospital Arrangements

While hospital affiliations are important to many physicians in that they affect their ability to deliver certain medical services, the extent to which specific contractual agreements with hospitals affects their incomes varies.

Table 2 presents the share and level of net income physicians derive from hospital agreements, according to the SMS findings.

The typical physician with a hospital contract reports that 62 percent of his/her income evolved from the arrangement. On average, this share represents approximately $59,500 in earnings.

Again, hospital contracts are most important for pathologists, who say they derive almost all (96%) of their income from these arrangements. Anesthesiologists and radiologists attribute 87 and 80 percent, respectively, of their net income to hospital agreements. In comparison, hospital contracts provide the smallest share of net income to general/family practitioners (40%) and to internists (40%).

Table 2

PERCENT NET INCOME DERIVED FROM HOSPITAL
ARRANGEMENTS, BY SPECIALTY

	Percent Income From Hospital Arrangement*	Average Net Income Derived From Arrangements
ALL PHYSICIANS**	62%	$59,500
Pathology	96	114,100
Anesthesiology	87	84,400
Radiology	80	108,900
Other Medical Specialties	70	55,600
Pediatrics	69	54,100
Psychiatry	56	40,800
General/Family Practice	40	(NA)
Internal Medicine	40	34,500

* This is the percent of net income that <u>physicians with arrangements</u> attribute to their financial contracts with the hospital.
** Too few observations are available to report income figures for the surgical classifications.
  "NA" denotes too few observations to report.

Types of Arrangements Physicians make with Hospitals

The two most common MD-hospital financial arrangements are salary and fee-for-service contracts. Approximately 60 percent of physicians with a hospital contract have a salary arrangement. One-third (33%) report they have a fee-for-service arrangement. Some physicians report arrangements which involve a percentage of the gross or net department billings as well.

Interspecialty variation in financial contracts is highlighted in Table 3. For example, 87 percent of the psychiatrists with contracts have salary arrangements while 16 percent report fee-for-service arrangements with hospitals (because some physicians have multiple arrangements, the sum of the percents exceed 100). In contrast, only 30 percent of the radiologists associated with hospitals are on salary, but 57 percent provide services on a fee-for-service basis.

Also, some physicians receive income from a percentage of gross or net billings. Twenty-one percent of pathologists with hospital contracts receive a percentage of gross department billings while three percent in this specialty receive a part of net billings. Thirteen percent of radiologists earn income from gross billings in the department as opposed to two percent from net billings. Generally, however, nine percent of all physicians with hospital contracts report earning a percentage of gross department billings as contrasted with only two percent who receive a percentage of net billings.

Table 3

TYPE OF CONTRACT FOR PHYSICIANS WITH HOSPITAL ARRANGEMENTS, BY SPECIALTY[1]

	Salary	Fee for Service	Percent of Gross Dept. Billings	Percent of Net Dept. Billings	Other[3]
ALL PHYSICIANS[2]	59%	33%	9%	2%	27%
General/Family Practice	60	27	10	3	19
Internal Medicine	58	45	4	0	22
Surgery	68	29	4	7	46
Psychiatry	87	16	6	3	24
Radiology	30	57	13	2	24
Pathology	53	21	21	3	19

1) The percentages reported in the table exceed 100 percent because some physicians have more than one financial arrangement.
2) Too few observations were available on obstetricians, pediatricians, and anesthesiologists to include these groups.
3) The most frequently encountered arrangements in this category include bonuses, leases, and a minimum guaranteed income, respectively.

AMBULATORY SURGERY*

Although some surgery has always been done on an ambulatory basis, free-standing ambulatory surgery centers and organized hospital-based ambulatory surgical programs are comparatively recent developments. Interest in these developments has been spurred by concern over the rising health care costs and findings which indicate that ambulatory surgery is less costly than inpatient surgery for appropriate procedures.

This report explores the following aspects of the practice of ambulatory surgery among physicians:

- the current extent of surgery on an ambulatory basis;

- recent changes in the amount of ambulatory surgery; and

- the types of locations used to perform such surgery.

The information reported is from the Socioeconomic Monitoring System survey conducted in the first quarter of 1982. The survey consisted of interviews with 1,268 physicians from a sample representative of the population of nonfederal patient care physicians, excluding residents.

Current Practice of Ambulatory Surgery

Ambulatory surgery is not uncommon. As shown in Table 1, over half of all surgical procedures are currently performed on an ambulatory basis. This includes nearly all surgical procedures performed by physicians in emergency medicine and three-quarters of those performed by general and family practitioners.

The smallest proportion of surgery that is done on an ambulatory basis, one-third, is among surgeons. The larger volume of surgery done by surgeons compared with other specialists, however, causes them to account for 40% of all ambulatory surgery.

The variation in the proportion of surgery done on an outpatient basis is probably due to differences in the mix of procedures typically performed by different specialists. Given the nature of their training, for example, surgical specialists are likely to more often perform complicated procedures that require post-operative inpatient care and

---

*Reprinted from SMS Report Volume 1, No. 4, May 1982.

Table 1

CURRENT EXTENT OF AMBULATORY SURGERY
AMONG PHYSICIANS WHO PERFORM SURGERY

Specialty	Percent of Surgery Performed on an Ambulatory Basis	Percent of Physicians Who Perform Any Ambulatory Surgery
ALL PHYSICIANS	51	82
General and Family Practice	75	82
Medical Specialties	57	71
Surgical Specialties	33	82
Emergency Medicine	98	100

supervision. General and family practitioners, on the other hand, are more likely to perform simple procedures that are suitable for an ambulatory approach. The data available do not make it possible, however, to distinguish among types of surgery.

In spite of the variation in the proportion of surgery done on an ambulatory basis, a widespread willingess by all physicians to perform surgery on an ambulatory basis, when it can be done safely and effectively, is evident.

Among surgeons and general and family practitioners who perform surgery, 82% do some on an ambulatory basis. In addition, all physicians in emergency medicine and 71% of medical specialtists who perform surgery use an ambulatory approach in some cases. Furthermore, large percentages of physicians in all major surgical subspecialties, in all census regions and in both solo and group practices do some surgery on an ambulatory basis.

Recent Changes in Ambulatory Surgery

As interest in ambulatory surgery has grown in the last two years, the extent of surgery performed on an ambulatory basis has increased (see Table 2). More than a third of all physicians who perform surgery have increased the amount they perform on an ambulatory basis in the last two years. The survey results also show that the amount of ambulatory surgery has unambiguously increased, even though 9% of physicians who perform surgery do less on an ambulatory basis than two years ago.

Table 2

PERCENT OF PHYSICIANS WHO PERFORM SURGERY
BY CURRENT AMOUNT OF AMBULATORY SURGERY
COMPARED TO TWO YEARS AGO

Specialty	More than 2 years ago	Same as 2 years ago	Less than 2 years ago
ALL PHYSICIANS	34	57	9
General and Family Practice	38	53	9
Medical Specialties	25	65	9
Surgical Specialties	37	55	8
Emergency Medicine	12	75	13

Among those increasing their amount of ambulatory surgery are nearly 40% of general and family practitioners and 25% of surgeons. The smaller proportion of physicians in emergency medicine increasing their amount of ambulatory surgery (12%) probably reflects the fact that so much of their surgery was already performed on an ambulatory basis two years ago that there was little room for increase.

Another indication of growth in the practice of ambulatory surgery is that 10% of physicians who currently perform ambulatory surgery performed no surgery on an outpatient basis two years ago. These physicians now perform 58% of their surgery on an ambulatory basis and account for 6% of the ambulatory surgery done by all physicians combined.

The recent increase in ambulatory surgery and the widespread willingness of physicians to perform appropriate procedures on an ambulatory basis suggest that ambualtory surgery is likely to become even more common as medical advances expand the types of surgery that can be performed on an outpatient basis.

Settings Used for Ambulatory Surgery

Table 3 suggests that the vast majority of ambulatory surgery is done in hospital-based ambulatory surgery centers and physicians' offices. Over 90% of physicians who perform ambulatory surgery do most of it in one of these two settings.

Although the development of free-standing ambulatory surgery centers has received much attention, such centers are still not commonly used. Only 7% of the physicians who do ambulatory surgery use ambulatory surgery centers at all; only 4% do most of their ambulatory surgery in these centers.

The degree to which different settings are used varies by specialty. While three-quarters of general and family practitioners perform most of their ambulatory surgery in their offices, 70% of surgeons use hospital-based centers most often. Medical specialists are more divided in the degree to which the two settings are most frequently used. The variation probably reflects the different types of facilities required for types of surgery typically performed by different specialties.

Table 3

SETTINGS USED BY PHYSICIANS WHO PERFORM AMBULATORY SURGERY

Specialty	Hospital-Based Ambulatory Surgery Center	Physician Office	Free-Standing Ambulatory Surgery Center
	Setting Used for Any Ambulatory Surgery: Percent of Physicians		
ALL PHYSICIANS	72	59	7
General and Family Practice	46	88	0
Medical Specialties	62	53	6
Surgical Specialties	87	50	10
Emergency Medicine	75	12	0
	Most Often Used Setting for Ambulatory Surgery: Percent of Physicians		
ALL PHYSICIANS	55	38	4
General and Family Practice	20	77	0
Medical Specialties	53	34	6
Surgical Specialties	69	24	4
Emergency Medicine	75	8	0

RECENT TRENDS IN PHYSICIAN LIABILITY CLAIMS AND INSURANCE EXPENSES*

The increasing frequency of physician liability claims and growth in size of awards led to a crisis in the physician liability insurance market in the mid-1970s. Physicians' premiums soared and many found themselves without insurance as the companies they had been dealing with withdrew from the market. By the end of 1976 physician liability insurance was accessible again, but the level of average premiums had risen 131 percent over 1973 levels.

This report summarizes physicians' experience with professional medical liability with special emphasis on:

● changes in the average annual incidence of claims since 1976 compared to earlier years; and

● changes in the distribution of medical liability insurance expenses among physicians since 1976.

The data are from the 1982 core survey of the AMA's Socioeconomic Monitoring System. The survey, conducted in the second quarter of 1982, consisted of interviews with 3,817 physicians from a sample representative of the population of nonfederal patient care physicians, excluding residents.

Recent Trends in Liability Claims

The incidence of claims is measured by the average number of claims per 100 physicians per year, as indicated in Table 1. The trend is clearly one of increasing vulnerability to claims for all physicians. This result holds true regardless of physicians' specialty, location, type of practice or sex. For all physicians, the average incidence of claims in recent years has doubled, increasing from 2.9 per 100 physicians per year prior to 1976 to 6.2 claims per year for the past five years.

Physicians' experience with liability claims has not been uniformly distributed across specialties. Obstetricians/gynecologists (OBGs), surgeons and radiologists are more susceptible to claims than other specialists. OBGs have had the highest average incidence of claims (14.0 per 100 physicians per year), as well as the greatest percentage increase in annual claims, since 1976. Psychiatrists and pediatricians have incurred claims at the lowest annual rates both prior to and after 1976.

---

*Reprinted from SMS Report Volume 1, No. 7, October 1982.

In addition to variation across specialties, current and past experiences with liability claims differ by type of practice and location. While solo physicians experienced an increase in claims of 93 percent, those in partnerships and groups experienced increases of 121 and 123 percent, respectively. Although solo and group physicians incurred claims at approximately the same rate prior to 1976, group physicians have experienced 19 percent more claims than physicians in solo practice in the last five years.

Physicians in the northeast and north central regions experienced a greater percentage increase in claims than those in other regions. In both regions the incidence of claims has increased by about 145 percent. At the other extreme, physicians in the west were least affected by the recent trend. The percentage increase for these physicians was only 52 percent.

Table 1

AVERAGE INCIDENCE OF PHYSICIAN LIABILITY CLAIMS
BY SPECIALTY, REGION, TYPE OF PRACTICE AND SEX

	Annual Claims per 100 Physicians	
	1976-1981	Prior to 1976
ALL PHYSICIANS	6.2	2.9
Specialty		
General/Family Practice	5.1	2.3
Internal Medicine	5.2	2.1
Surgical Specialty	9.2	4.5
Pediatrics	3.6	1.5
Obstetrics/Gynecology	14.0	5.3
Radiology	5.9	3.1
Psychiatry	1.9	1.0
Anesthesiology	5.2	2.6
Other	3.7	2.1
Region		
Northeast	7.6	3.1
North Central	6.2	2.5
South	5.2	2.3
West	6.4	4.2
Type of Practice		
Solo	5.8	3.0
Partnership	7.5	3.4
Group	6.9	3.1
Other	4.9	1.9
Sex		
Male	6.5	3.0
Female	3.2	2.3

Female physicians have been less seriously affected by the growth in claims since 1976 than their male counterparts. Prior to 1976, women incurred about 25 percent fewer claims than men. However, since 1976 female physicians have reported only 50 percent as many claims as male physicians.

Physician Liability Insurance Expenses

A major concern with the trend in claims is its potential impact on liability insurance premiums and, ultimately, the price of physician services.

SMS data show that 1981 expenditures on liability insurance are positively related to the recent claims experience of physicians. Physicians paying $4,000 or less in 1981 experienced an average of 5.0 claims per 100 physicians per year since 1976, while those paying at least $20,000 experienced over 18.0 claims per 100 physicians annually on average.

Given the positive association between recent claims and premium expenses, it might be expected that the increase in claims since 1976 would have caused an upward shift in the distribution of premium expenses between 1976 and 1981. Table 2 shows how the distribution of premiums among physicians actually changed from 1976 to 1981.

The data indicate that 63 percent of all physicians paid $4,000 or less for liability insurance in 1981 compared with 66 percent in 1976. This suggests that for a large percentage of the physician population liability insurance expenses have not increased substantially. The observed trend in premiums does not appear to adequately reflect the increase in claims frequency. In large part, this may be due to the fact that a significant number of insurers now offer claims-made instead of occurrence coverage.

The primary distinction between a claims-made policy and an occurrence policy is that the former does not protect the physician against future liabilities. In other words, while an occurence policy covers all claims resulting from incidents that happen in a particular year regardless of when the claim is made, a claims-made policy only insures against claims resulting from incidents reported in the current policy year and in preceding years for which a claims-made policy was in effect. Therefore, a claims-made policy is initially less expensive than an occurrence policy. However, as exposure increases over time, the premiums for claims-made policies will mature to a level close to that of occurrence coverage.

Despite the small increase overall, premiums show a significant upward shift within certain specialties. In 1976 only 4 percent of OBGs paid premiums of $20,000 or more. By 1981, that percentage had increased to 16 percent. The greatest increase in the percent of physicians paying more than $4,000 in premiums occurred among radiologists. This group grew from 25 percent of radiologists in 1976 to 44 percent in 1981.

If the incidence of claims and severity of awards continues to grow as it has in the past five years, it is likely that liability premiums will increase sharply in the near future. Since the increase in the incidence of claims is not occurring uniformly among all physicians, rising liability premiums will impose greater hardships on certain segments of the physician population.

Table 2

PERCENTAGE DISTRIBUTION OF PHYSICIANS
BY LIABILITY INSURANCE EXPENSES*, 1981 AND 1976**

Specialty	Year	0 to $4,000	$5,000 to 9,000	$10,000 to 19,000	$20,000 and over
ALL PHYSICIANS	1981	63.1%	21.9%	11.4%	3.6%
	1976	65.6	20.7	11.0	2.6
General/Family Practice	1981	72.7	17.4	3.7	1.2
	1976	82.3	12.7	3.1	1.8
Internal Medicine	1981	76.9	19.2	2.7	1.2
	1976	87.3	11.1	0.9	0.6
Surgery	1981	33.9	34.7	25.3	6.1
	1976	34.6	37.3	23.6	4.5
Pediatrics	1976	93.1	5.6	0.4	0.9
	1981	83.8	13.1	3.0	0.0
Obstetrics/ Gynecology	1981	30.3	25.9	27.7	16.1
	1976	24.4	41.6	30.2	3.8
Radiology	1981	56.4	34.6	7.3	1.8
	1976	75.3	14.9	9.8	0.0
Psychiatry	1981	95.0	3.6	1.4	0.0
	1976	98.1	1.5	0.4	0.0
Anesthesiology	1981	35.5	30.3	26.3	7.9
	1976	19.7	36.9	29.9	13.4
Other	1981	83.5	13.0	2.6	0.9
	1976	82.0	13.0	3.8	1.3

---

*Expense data reported for self-employed physicians only. The liability insurance expense data has been rounded to the nearest thousand and grouped for purposes of presentation.
**1976 data are from the AMA Eleventh Periodic Survey of Physicians.

CHANGES IN THE USE OF PROCEDURES AMONG PHYSICIANS*

The practice of medicine is constantly evolving. Treatments and procedures are continually being developed or modified in ways that advance the state of the art. These changes in medical practice may have a number of effects on the health care marketplace. They may improve the quality of care. They may also increase the amount of society's resources utilized in the delivery of health care. On a more practical level, changes may be required in current reimbursement methods in order to reflect the expense or technical requirements of new procedures.

It is therefore important to examine both the impact of new diagnostic and therapeutic procedures on practicing physicians, and the nature of the process used by physicians in deciding whether to adopt these procedures. This report uses data from AMA's Socioeconomic Monitoring System (SMS) to investigate three important aspects of this process:

- the extent to which physicians adopt new procedures and drop old ones;

- the sources used by physicians to learn about new procedures; and

- the extent to which physicians decide not to adopt new procedures, and their reasons for doing so.

The data are from the first quarter SMS 1982 survey, which contains responses from 1,268 non-federal patient care physicians, excluding residents. The survey response rate was 66.8 percent.

Changes in the Use of Procedures

The most fundamental aspect of this issue is the frequency with which physicians modify their methods of practice based on advances in medical science. Thus, in the SMS survey physicians were asked whether during the past twelve months they performed any new diagnostic or therapeutic procedures that reflected recent advances in medical knowledge or technology. (The use of new prescription drugs was explicitly excluded.) Physicians were also asked whether they dropped any procedures from their normal office routine during the past twelve months.

The response to these questions, presented in Table 1, indicates a substantial level of adoption of new procedures by practicing physicians. For all physicians, 37 percent adopted new procedures and 14 percent

---

*Reprinted from SMS Report Volume 1, No. 9, December 1982.

Table 1

PERCENTAGE OF PHYSICIANS ADOPTING AND DISCONTINUING PROCEDURES

	Adopting New Procedures	Discontinuing Procedures
ALL PHYSICIANS*	37%	14%
General and Family Practice	19	7
Medical Specialties	36	13
Surgery	46	15
Obstetrics/Gynecology	18	6
Radiology	62	43

*Includes other specialties not reported separately.

dropped procedures in the past year. With the exception of obstetrics/gynecology, physicians in the specialty groups were more likely to adopt new procedures than general and family practitioners. This finding conforms with the expectation that innovations in the science of medicine are more likely to be adopted, at least initially, by physicians working in more technologically oriented areas.

A further question asked physicians who had dropped procedures whether these procedures were replaced by new ones. Seventy-seven percent of the physicians responding indicated that at least one of the dropped procedures was replaced by a new procedure.

The picture which emerges from these data is one of an increasingly more complicated and sophisticated practice of medicine. For all specialty groups shown, the percentage of physicians adopting new procedures is substantially greater than the percentage of physicians who dropped procedures. This differential implies that the array of procedures utilized by each specialty is increasing. For radiology in particular, the rapid rate of technological change is reflected in both the adoption of new procedures and the abandonment of old ones.

Sources of Information on New Procedures

Physicians learn about new procedures through a variety of methods. Each of these may have certain advantages relative to the others. For example, professional meetings may provide the type of interaction which physicians can use to determine how well procedures fit into their specific practices. On the other hand, articles in medical journals may provide more detailed analytical and clinical information in a format conducive to careful consideration of the merits of a new procedure.

Given the growing complexity of medical practice, it is important to determine how physicians learn about new procedures. Physicians in the

Table 2

PERCENTAGE DISTRIBUTION OF
MOST IMPORTANT SOURCES OF INFORMATION ON NEW PROCEDURES

	Medical Journals	Professional Meetings	Discussions w/other Physicians	Government Technology Assessments	Other
ALL PHYSICIANS*	41%	43%	11%	0%	5%
General and Family Practice	36	40	15	0	9
Medical Specialties	51	37	9	0	3
Surgery	36	53	8	1	2
Obstetrics/ Gynecology	27	64	9	0	0
Radiology	48	38	7	0	7

*Includes other specialties not reported separately.

SMS survey were therefore asked about their sources of information on new procedures. Over 95 percent of physicians utilize medical journals; professional meetings, conferences, or continuing education courses; and discussions with other physicians to learn about new procedures. However, only 20 percent use technology assessments provided by government agencies, and only 25 percent utilize other sources.

Further insight into the sources of information on new procedures can be gained by analyzing which sources physicians considered to be the most important, as presented in Table 2. For all specialty groups shown, medical journals and professional meetings are considered the most important sources of information on new procedures by the vast majority of physicians. Physicians in the medical specialties and radiology placed slightly more emphasis on medical journals, while those in surgery and obstetrics/gynecology placed more emphasis on professional meetings. Although discussions with other physicians are utilized by physicians to learn about new procedures, it is evident from Table 2 that most do not consider these discussions to be the most important source. Government technology assessments and other sources play an even smaller role.

Reasons for Not Adopting New Procedures

Physicians do not adopt every new procedure that might be relevant to their practice. Indeed, 55 percent of all physicians indicated that over the past year they learned about some relevant new diagnostic or therapeutic procedure that they chose not to adopt. Among specialty groups, the response ranged from 33 percent of general and family practitioners learning about a new procedure they chose not to adopt, to 72 percent for radiologists.

Table 3

REASONS FOR NOT ADOPTING NEW PROCEDURES

	Insufficient Information About Safety and Effectiveness	Necessary Equipment Not Available	Procedure Already Performed at Facility In Area	Costs Too Great Relative to Patient Benefits
ALL PHYSICIANS*	59%	62%	44%	54%
General and Family Practice	52	91	78	61
Medical Specialites	63	62	46	52
Surgery	68	48	36	46
Obstetrics/Gynecology	64	68	32	81
Radiology	43	81	29	38

*Includes other specialties not reported separately.

A number of factors enter into the decision whether or not to adopt a new procedure. Physicians who indicated they had chosen not to adopt a procedure were asked whether four specific considerations (shown in Table 3) had any impact on their decisions.

Most physicians indicated that more than one reason played a role in their decision not to adopt a new procedure. General and family practitioners most often indicated that the necessary equipment or facilities for performing the procedure were not available, and that the procedure was already performed at a hospital or other medical facility in the area. These physicians apparently forego some procedures relevant to their practice in favor of other specialists who would be expected to perform the procedure more frequently.

Concern about the cost implications of new procedures is manifested in at least two dimensions. Over half of all physicians indicated that one reason for not adopting a procedure was the possibility that its costs would exceed the benefits to their patients.

An even larger percentage stated that the unavailability of the necessary equipment was also a factor. One likely reason for this response is a perception on the part of the physician that purchasing the equipment would not be financially sound. For example, financial considerations are no doubt an important reason why radiologists most often cited the lack of equipment as the reason why a procedure was not adopted. Many advances in this field (such as CAT scanners and nuclear magnetic resonance machines) are capital-intensive and very expensive. Thus, cost considerations are a key element in physicians' decisions regarding the adoption of new procedures.

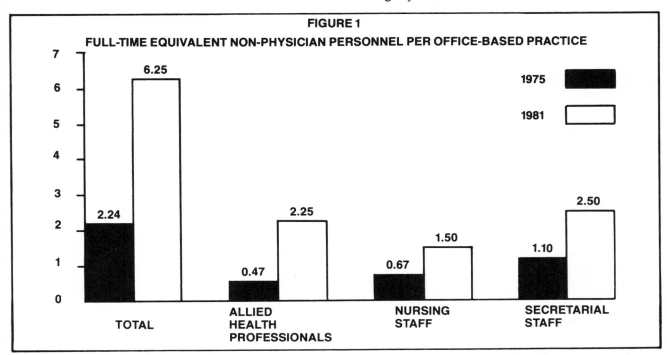

FIGURE 1
FULL-TIME EQUIVALENT NON-PHYSICIAN PERSONNEL PER OFFICE-BASED PRACTICE

PHYSICIAN UTILIZATION OF ALLIED HEALTH PROFESSIONALS*

In the last two decades there has been a dramatic increase in the number and kinds of non-physician personnel -- allied health professionals, nurses, and secretarial staff -- employed by physicians in their practices. This trend has been particularly acute for allied health professionals (AHPs).

Four major factors account for these events:

● rapid advances in medical technology, which expand the kinds of medical services that physicians can provide, but which increasingly require delegation of tasks;

● the growth in the number and size of group practices, which can benefit from the advantages of larger scale in utilizing non-physician personnel;

● an ever-increasing concern about cost containment and cost-effective strategies for delivering medical care; and

● the economic forces resulting from greater competition in all elements of the health care sector.

*Reprinted from SMS Report Volume 1, No. 10, December 1982.

This report examines the utilization of non-physician personnel (especially AHPs) in physicians' practices, including:

- the growth in the number of AHPs and other non-physician personnel in medical practices; and

- the consequences of physician employment of AHPs.

The information presented is from two sources: the 1982 SMS core survey and the 1975 Periodic Survey of Physicians (PSP). Although the SMS sample (n=3817) encompasses all U.S. nonfederal patient-care physicians (excluding residents), those physicians practicing in settings other than the office were excluded to permit comparison with the office-based sample (n=5288) of physicians surveyed by PSP.

Non-Physician Personnel per Practice

The growth in the number of non-physician personnel employed by physicians can be demonstrated in two dimensions: employees per practice and employees per physician. Figure 1 shows that the average office-based practice employs nearly three times the number of non-physician personnel as it did in 1975: the number of full-time equivalent personnel per practice increased from 2.24 in 1975 to 6.25 in 1981.*

Increases in the average number of health-related employees and office personnel offer evidence that the structure of medical practice has been changing for physicians. The doubling of nursing and secretarial staff since 1975 indicates that additional personnel are required to handle the numerous procedural and administrative tasks inherent in today's practice environment, particularly in group practices.

More dramatic is the almost five-fold increase in the number of allied health professionals per office-based practice during this period, from 0.47 per practice in 1975 to 2.25 in 1981. This growth reflects, at least in part, the gains to specialization in the delivery of medical care attributable to advances in medical technology and the increasing prevalence of group practices. That is, physician practices are able to increase their productivity by assigning appropriate preparatory and ancillary tasks to these personnel.

---

* For ease of presentation, non-physician employees were aggregated into three categories: allied health professionals (including physicians' assistants, x-ray technicians, medical laboratory technicians, respiratory therapists and technicians, physicial therapists, radiation therapists, EEG technologists, occupational therapists, perfusionists, and medical assistants); nursing staff (registered nurses, licensed practical nurses, and nurse practitioners); and secretarial staff (secretaries, receptionists, and clerks).

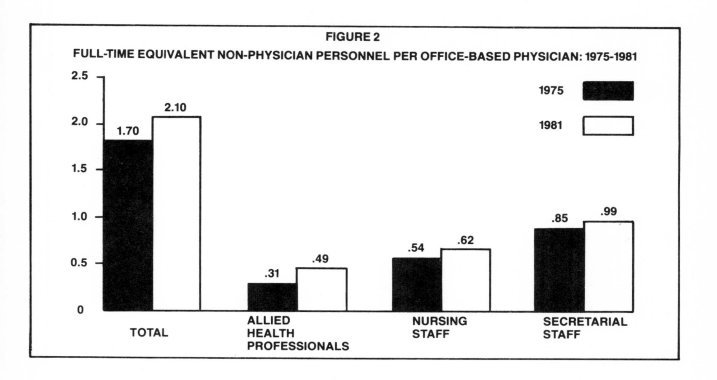

FIGURE 2

FULL-TIME EQUIVALENT NON-PHYSICIAN PERSONNEL PER OFFICE-BASED PHYSICIAN: 1975-1981

Non-Physician Personnel per Physician

The trends in utilization of non-physician personnel are also evident in the changing number and composition of non-physician personnel with whom individual physicians work. In this context, Figure 2 presents the number of full-time equivalent personnel employed per physician in 1975 and 1981.

In 1975, office-based physicians worked with an average of 1.7 non-physician personnel. By 1981, this figure had increased to 2.1. By far the largest percentage increase occurred in the allied health professionals category, which rose from 0.31 AHPs per physician in 1975 to 0.49 in 1981, an increase of 58 percent. The expanded utilization of AHPs clearly demonstrates one way in which physicians are responding to the increasingly complex nature of medical care delivery.

Another way of describing this change is by multiplying the numbers in Figure 2 by 100. From this perspective, 49 full-time AHPs were employed per 100 physicians in 1981, 18 per 100 physicians more than in 1975. The 1981 level can be disaggregated into the component professions of AHPs (although not shown in the figure). Thus, in 1981, every 100 patient-care office-based physicians accounted for the employment of 20 laboratory technicians, 16 medical assistants, 7 physicians' assistants, two x-ray technicians, and one each of respiratory therapists, physical therapists, radiation therapists, and EEG technologists. (Comparable data from 1975 are not available.)

Table 1

CONSEQUENCES OF PHYSICIAN EMPLOYMENT OF SELECTED AHPS, 1981

Practice Characteristics	Employment of Nurse Practitioners or Physicians' Assistants	
	None	Some
Patient Visits Per Hour*	3.2	3.9
Patient Visits Per Week*	86.2	103.1
Physicians' Weeks Worked Per Year	46.6	46.7
Physicians' Net Income* ($000)	93.7	106.0
Fee -- office visit for established patient	$23.19	$22.45

*Differences in values are significant at the 1% level.

Consequences of Physician Employment of Selected AHPs

Figures 1 and 2 indicate significant changes in physicians' utilization of non-physician employees in recent years. It is also important to examine the impact these personnel changes have had on physicians' practices and on the production of cost-effective medical care. For instance, if physicians who delegate appropriate tasks are more productive, then evidence of these productivity differences should appear in various aspects of their practices.

Table 1 presents the means of five selected practice characteristics for physicians who employ some AHPs compared to those physicians who use none of these AHPs. Physicians were categorized according to whether they work with nurse practitioners (NPs) or physicians' assistants (PAs); these employees are those most likely to provide preparatory or ancillary tasks otherwise performed by the physician. Visits per hour represents one measure of productivity of physicians in the delivery of medical care. Patient visits per week and the average number of weeks worked per year by physicians measure the total output of services. Physicians' net income is included to demonstrate revenue gains associated with higher productivity. Finally, the fee for an office visit of an established patient reflects the average cost of producing medical services.

As shown in the table, physicians who do not work with NPs or PAs provide fewer patient visits than those who do, both on an hourly and weekly basis. Since the two groups of physicians exhibit similar work years, the productivity differences seem to hold on an annual basis as well. The greater output of services by physicians who employ NPs or PAs results in higher average earnings for these physicians. Finally, the similarity of fees for an office visit for an established patient indicates that physician employment of NPs or PAs does not necessarily raise the average cost of medical care to patients.

PHYSICIAN-HOSPITAL RELATIONS*

Over the past 20 years, the role of hospitals in the practice of medicine has increased dramatically. From an institution established primarily for the care of indigent patients, the hospital today is an essential part of the delivery of modern medical care.

Because the physician occupies such a prominent position in the delivery of quality hospital care, considerable attention has focused on the nature of physician-hospital relations. In light of the growing number of new physicians who will be seeking hospital privileges and the increasing likelihood that hospitals will restrict medical staff appointments, the importance of physician-hospital relations will probably intensify. Two aspects of particular interest have been in the areas of hospital medical directors and governing boards. Both have a significant impact on physician-hospital relations and, ultimately, physician satisfaction with hospital medical services.

This report summarizes selected aspects of physician-hospital relations with special emphasis on:

- hospital admitting privileges;
- medical staffing and department closure;
- full-time medical directors and physicians' satisfaction; and
- governing body representation and physicians' interests.

The data are from the AMA's third quarter 1982 Socioeconomic Monitoring System (SMS) survey. The SMS survey includes interviews with 1,247 physicians from a sample representative of the population of all non-federal patient care physicians excluding residents. The survey response was 61 percent.

Hospital Admitting Privileges

Hospital admitting privileges are crucial to the medical practice of many physicians. As Table 1 reveals, an average of 91.4 percent of patient care physicians in 1982 indicate that they have hospital admitting privileges. Among the major specialties, medical and surgical specialties have the highest level of physicians with admitting privileges (97.4% and 97.0% respectively). In contrast, only 70.5 percent of physicians in the other specialty (OS) group reveal they have admitting privileges.

---

*Reprinted from SMS Report Volume 1, No. 11, December 1982.

Compared to 1977 information obtained from the AMA's Twelfth Periodic Survey of Physicians (PSP), it appears that physician admitting privileges have declined 2.7 percent in the past five years. The major portion of the decline results from the 11.4 percent drop in admitting privileges for physicians in the other specialty group.

Table 1

CHANGING PATTERNS IN HOSPITAL ADMITTING PRIVILEGES, 1977 AND 1982

| | Percentage of Physicians with Admitting Privileges | | Change in the Percentage |
	1977*	1982**	
ALL SPECIALTIES	94.1%	91.4%	−2.7%
General and Family Practice	92.7	90.5	−2.2
Medical Specialties	97.7	97.4	−0.3
Surgical Specialties	98.9	97.0	−1.9
Other Specialties***	81.9	70.5	−11.4

*Source: AMA's Twelfth Periodic Survey of Physicians.
**To make SMS data comparable to PSP, physicians with a plurality of hours in non-office based activities are excluded from this column.
***Anesthesiologists, Pathologists, and Radiologists are excluded because they generally do not admit patients.

Medical Staffs and Department Closure

The potential for competition among hospitals as well as competition between a hospital and its medical staff raises important questions about hospital staffing and department closure. Table 2 indicates that the majority of physicians (91.3%) feel that their medical staff has a sufficient number of physicians. General and family practitioners are the least likely (88.4%) to perceive their medical staff as having a sufficient number of physicians, while physicians in surgical specialties are most likely (92.4%).

On average, 17.4 percent of all physicians have admitting privileges at hospitals which have departments or clinical services that are closed to appointments of new, qualified medical practitioners. General and family practitioners (6.4%) are less likely than the other types of specialties to have admitting privileges at hospitals with closed departments. Physicians located in the northeast census region are most likely (23.6%) to have admission privileges in a hospital with closed staffing while only 15.2 percent of physicians in the north central region report they practice in hospitals with closed departments.

Table 2

MEDICAL STAFFING AND DEPARTMENT CLOSURE,
BY SPECIALTY AND REGION

	Sufficient Medical Staff	Departments Closed to New Appointments
ALL PHYSICIANS	91.3%	17.4%
Specialty		
General and Family Practice	88.4	6.4
Medical Specialties	91.6	22.4
Surgical Specialties	92.4	17.8
Other Specialties	91.8	20.2
Region		
Northeast	93.5	23.6
North Central	89.5	15.2
South	89.7	15.9
West	93.5	16.7

Medical Directors and Physicians' Satisfaction

Hospitals vary widely in their organizational structure. As Table 3 indicates, 49.3 percent of all physicians with admitting privileges admit most of their patients to hospitals with a full-time hospital medical director. General and family practitioners who have hospital privileges are least likely (35.6%) to work in a hospital which has a full-time medical director, while physicians in the OS category (57.9%) are most likely to work in a hospital which has a full-time medical director.

On the whole, 85.1 percent of all physicians feel that the medical director represents the interest of the medical staff and this response is fairly uniform over the various specialties. General and family practitioners are the least likely to view the medical director as strengthening physician-hospital relationships (79.7%), although they are similar to other physicians in their feeling that the medical director provides effective organizational services (92.3%).

The presence of a medical director varies widely among the census regions. In the northeast region, 63.1 percent of the physicians interviewed report that they had admitting privileges at hospitals with full-time medical directors. In contrast, only 39.5 percent of the physicians in the south report a full-time medical director.

Physicians located in the northeastern and southern regions appear similar (90.1% and 90.7% respectively) in their feeling that the medical director strengthens the physician-hospital relationship. Physicians in the north central and western regions are less likely (81.1% and 82.7% respectively) to view the medical director as strengthening physician-hospital relationships when compared to physicians in the other two regions.

-33-

Table 3

FULL-TIME MEDICAL DIRECTORS: PHYSICIAN SATISFACTION
BY SPECIALTY AND REGION

	Percentage of Physicians with a Full-Time Medical Director	Director		
		Represents Physician Interests	Strengthens Physician Hospital Relationship	Provides Effective Organizational Services
ALL PHYSICIANS	49.3%	85.1%	86.3%	91.0%
Specialty				
General and Family Practice	35.6	86.2	79.7	92.3
Medical Specialties	52.6	85.0	86.6	88.4
Surgical Specialties	48.2	81.2	85.0	89.0
Other Specialties	57.9	89.1	90.4	95.5
Region				
Northeast	63.1	81.1	90.1	90.8
North Central	53.2	84.3	81.1	91.2
South	39.5	88.6	90.7	93.8
West	47.3	86.4	82.7	87.9

Governing Body Representation and Physician Interests

Physician representation on hospital governing bodies is an effective method for strengthening physician-hospital relations and assuring physician input in the hospital decision making process. In Table 4, the majority of physicians (88.4%) reveal that their hospital has at least one physician on the governing board. Furthermore, 89.8 percent of the respondents reveal that the physicians on the governing body adequately represent their interests. Physicians in general and family practice are most likely to report (93.8%) that physicians on the governing board represent their interests, while physicians in surgical specialties are least likely (84.7%).

Table 4
Governing Body Representation: Physician Satisfaction by Specialty

	Percentage of Physicians with a Physician On Governing Board	Physician Represents Medical Staff Interest
ALL PHYSICIANS	88.4%	89.8%
Specialty		
General and Family Practice	78.9	93.8
Medical Specialties	89.4	91.9
Surgical Specialties	90.6	84.7
Other Specialties	91.9	91.8

THE IMPACT OF THE 1981–82 RECESSION ON MEDICAL PRACTICE*

The recession that began in mid–1981 and continued through December 1982 was marked by the highest unemployment rates since 1940 and reductions in real (that is, inflation-adjusted) gross national product to 1979 levels. This economic environment may have had a number of effects on physicians and their practices. This report explores:

- changes in weekly patient visits and net practice income over the course of the recession; and

- physician efforts to provide care for free or at reduced rates for patients who lost health insurance due to unemployment or who lost Medicaid coverage due to program cutbacks.

The data are from the initial SMS survey in fourth quarter 1981 and from surveys thereafter through fourth quarter 1982. Over 1200 physicians from a representative sample of the population of nonfederal, patient care physicians were surveyed in each quarter.

Trends in Practice Indicators

A recession can affect physicians' practices in a number of ways. Reductions in real income and increased unemployment among patients may decrease their utilization of physician services. In addition, diminished purchasing power can increase unpaid physician billings. This section examines trends in average weekly patient visits and average practice net income from mid–1981 through the end of 1982 in order to assess the effect of the recession on physicians' economic well-being.

Average patient visits per week for all patient-care physicians did indeed fall from the fourth quarter of 1981 to the first half of 1982, as reported in Table 1. However, this decline was more than offset by increases in patient visits from the first half to second half of 1982. This increase occurred in spite of a deepening of the recession in this period. Overall, average patient visits increased by about 1 visit per week for all physicians during 1982.

Changes in patient visits varied by specialty. Weekly visits fell by about five visits per week for general and family practice physicians and by about one visit per week for surgical specialties from the fourth quarter of 1981 to the second half of 1982. Physicians in medical spe-

---

*Reprinted from SMS Report Volume 2, No. 2, February 1982.

Table 1

AVERAGE PATIENT VISITS PER WEEK*
4th QUARTER 1981 - 2nd HALF 1982

	4th Qtr 1981	1st Half 1982	2nd Half 1982
ALL PHYSICIANS**	132.6	130.2	134.1
General and Family Practice	163.3	160.3	158.2
Medical Specialties	121.4	124.2	126.4
Surgical Specialties	126.4	119.4	124.8

*Includes office visits, visits on hospital rounds, emergency room and outpatient visits, and other visits.

**Includes all specialties except for Psychiatry, Anesthesiology, Radiology, and Pathology.

cialties, however, experienced an increase of about five visits per week on average. These changes represent at most only a 4 percent change in patient visits per week. We can conclude, therefore, that utilization of physician services remained relatively stable over the period considered. Extended insurance coverage may be one explanation for the stable utilization rates.

On average, patients did not reduce their utilization of medical care even as the state of the economy deteriorated. It is undeniable that some individuals deferred visits to a physician because they were unemployed, faced the prospect of unemployment, or were otherwise affected by the recession. Nevertheless, it appears that individuals and families overall reduced their expenditures for other goods and services in order to ensure the maintenance of their health care.

Since patient visits remained quite stable, we should expect that physicians' net practice incomes were not adversely affected by the recession. Data reported in Table 2 support this claim. Physicians in all four specialty groups actually experienced an increase in quarterly practice income, net of expenses but before taxes, over the period examined. For all specialties, there was a large increase between the second half of 1981 and the first half of 1982. SMS data suggest that these increases in income occurred because of an increase in average fees paid for physicians' services over this period. Income trends moderated from the first half to the second half of 1982, especially for general and family practitioners and surgical specialists.

Physicians in the North Central region, one of the areas hardest hit by the recession, maintained their income positions relative to physicians in the South and Northwest. These three regions experienced virtually identical relative increases in quarterly income from the second half of 1981 to the second half of 1982. Physicians in the West had the

Table 2

AVERAGE QUARTERLY NET INCOME
2nd HALF 1981 – 2nd HALF 1982

	2nd Half 1981	1st Half 1982	2nd Half 1982
ALL PHYSICIANS	$22,600	$26,200	$27,300
SPECIALTY			
General and Family Practice	17,500	20,300	20,100
Medical Specialties	19,600	23,600	24,800
Surgical Specialties	27,900	33,200	33,100
Other Specialties	22,800	25,400	27,600
REGION			
Northeast	19,400	23,600	23,600
North Central	22,600	25,500	28,000
South	24,000	28,400	29,500
West	24,000	26,200	26,500

smallest increase in quarterly income, both in relative and absolute terms. This result cannot be explained by the recession, since the West was only minimally affected by the depressed economy. Competition among providers may be more intense in the West, limiting increases in income.

Though there is little evidence of a national effect of the recession on physicians, it is important to note that some physicians may not be doing as well as practice indicators suggest. Effects of the recession in localized areas, such as specific cities or states, are not readily observed in small samples designed to be representative of the profession as a whole. Thus, individual physicians may indeed be experiencing some difficulties even though this is not reflected in the national average.

Impact of Economy on Medical Practice

Although overall practice indicators show little direct economic impact of the recession on physicians, the state of the economy is indeed having some effect on medical practice. There is considerable evidence that physicians have responded to the special needs of those patients who were adversely affected by the recession. The SMS survey conducted in the fourth quarter of 1982 inquired as to physicians' efforts to assist needy patients. Table 3 reports the results.

Seventy-nine percent of physicians surveyed stated that in the previous month (September 1982) they had treated patients who had lost health insurance due to unemployment. In addition, 35 percent responded that they had treated patients who had lost Medicaid coverage due to program cutbacks.

Table 3

IMPACT OF THE ECONOMY ON MEDICAL PRACTICE

IMPACT OF RECESSION

Percent of Physicians Treating Some Patients Who Lost Health
Insurance Due to Unemployment   79%

Of Those Physicians Treating Some Patients Who Lost Benefits:

   Percent Providing Free or Reduced Fee Care   71

   Average Percent Reduction in Physician Billings   6

IMPACT OF MEDICAID CUTBACKS

Percent of Physicians Treating Some Patients Who Lost Medicaid
Coverage Due to Program Cutbacks   35

Of Those Physicians Treating Some Patients Who Lost Benefits:

   Percent Providing Some Free or Reduced Fee Care   55

   Average Percent Reduction in Physician Billings   5

FAIR SHARE PROGRAM PARTICIPATION

Percent of Physicians Participating in Organized Fair
Share Programs   10

Physicians have been assisting their needy patients through numerous voluntary actions. Of those physicians surveyed who were treating unemployed patients without health insurance, 71 percent provided at least some care for free or at reduced rates. Fifty-five percent of those with patients who lost Medicaid benefits said that they have provided similar assistance to patients so affected. Furthermore, 10 percent of physicians surveyed donated their services to some type of "fair-share" program. These programs are organized by community leaders and state medical societies to provide health care for those who have lost their primary source of income but do not qualify for government assistance.

These efforts to aid the needy have affected the billings of physicians. Those providing free or reduced fee care to the unemployed experienced on average a six percent decline in their potential billings in September 1982. A five percent decline, on average, resulted for those physicians providing similar assistance to those who lost Medicaid coverage. Fifteen percent of those physicians assisting the needy had reductions in physician billings of over 10 percent. Physicians from all specialty and geographic areas have volunteered their services in response to the special needs of their patients.

PHYSICIAN RESPONSES TO COMPETITION*

Competition facing physicians is increasing rapidly. Several factors have contributed to this trend. Rising health care costs have resulted in greater cost-consciousness among purchasers of health care services. The number of physicians has increased at a rate four times faster than the population since 1970. At the same time, the costs of practicing medicine have been rising sharply. These pressures are making it more difficult for some physicians to attract and retain patients and are heightening physician concern over the cost-effectiveness of their practices.

This report focuses on physician responses in adjusting to a more competitive environment. The types of responses examined include:

- changes in characteristics of practice services, and

- adoption of new marketing strategies and techniques.

The report is based on information from the 4th quarter 1982 survey of the Socioeconomic Monitoring System (SMS). The survey included interviews with 1,215 physicians from a sample representative of the population of all non-federal patient care physicians excluding residents. The survey response rate was 63%.

Changes in Characteristics of Practice Services

Three aspects of practice services in which changes might be expected, in response to competition, are: the number of housecalls made, the number of scheduled week-end and evening office hours, and the number of non-physician personnel employed by physicians. An increased number of housecalls and scheduled week-end and evening office hours are approaches to increasing the accessibility of a physician's services and alleviating problems in attracting patients. Increased employment of non-physician personnel may reflect two different types of responses to competition. First, it may indicate an effort to improve practice productivity and reduce the cost of services delivered. It may also reflect an expansion of the range of services provided by physicians in their offices in an effort to attract larger patient bases.

The changes that have occurred in these three aspects of practice services in the last two years are shown in Table 1. Only 8% of physicians are making more housecalls and only 5% are scheduling more hours on week-ends and in the evening. Slightly greater percentages of all

---

*Reprinted from SMS Report Volume 2, No. 3, June 1983.

Table 1

CHANGES IN CHARACTERISTICS OF PRACTICE SERVICE
IN THE LAST TWO YEARS

Current Number Compared to 2 years Ago	Percent of Physicians by Years of Practice*		
	All Physicians	10 Years or less	Over 10 Years
Housecalls per month			
More	8	11	7
Same	77	80	75
Fewer	14	9	17
Hours scheduled for evening			
More	5	12	2
Same	85	76	88
Fewer	10	12	9
FTE non-physician employees under physician's supervision			
More	22	34	18
Same	67	59	71
Fewer	11	8	12

*Percents may not add to 100 due to rounding. Percents are accurate within ± 3%.

physicians are actually providing fewer of each of these services than two years ago. Two factors may account for the apparent lack of response to competitive pressure in these dimensions of practice services. First, there may not be an effective patient demand for these services. Hospital emergency services may be viewed as satisfactory substitutes in most instances for physician housecalls or office hours outside the normal work week. Second, physicians may not regard the benefits of these services as warranting the cost of their time when compared with other methods for responding to competitive pressures.

A more evident impact of competition is suggested by the increased employment of non-physician personnel by 22% of physicians in the last two years. At the same time, only 11% of physicians have reduced the size of their non-physician staff.

Since physicians with more years of practice generally have better developed practices, they may be expected to experience less of an impact from competitive pressures than younger physicians. This expectation is confirmed by the larger percentage of physicians with 10 or fewer years of practice that are making changes in characteristics of their services compared with those with more practice years. The response by younger physicians is particularly strong in the hiring of non-physician employees. While 34% of young physicians are making greater use of non-physician staff than two years ago, only 18% of more experienced physicians have responded to competition in this manner.

Adoption of Marketing Strategies and Techniques

Although less commonly employed in the medical sector than in other sectors of the economy in the past, marketing strategies and techniques may be more frequently used by physicians to identify patient needs and attract patients as the competitive pressures increase. The SMS survey asked physicians about eight particular marketing strategies or techniques they may have used in the last five years to learn about the extent to which this type of response to competition is already occurring. The different marketing strategies and techniques asked about are listed in Table 2.

Altogether, 40% of physicians have employed at least one of the marketing approaches. The most common measure has been studies of community demographics to assess patient needs. Of physicians reporting, 27% have made such studies in the last five years. In addition, 13% of physicians have used surveys to learn about patient satisfaction with various aspects of their practices, 11% have opened satellite clinics and 9% have advertised their practice in the media. Smaller percentages of physicians have adopted the other four approaches -- initiating a patient newsletter, hiring a marketing consultant, developing marketing plan for their practice and locating their practice in a non-traditional setting, such as a storefront or shopping center.

Table 2

MARKETING STRATEGIES AND TECHNIQUES EMPLOYED BY PHYSICIANS
IN THE LAST FIVE YEARS

Strategy or Technique Employed in Last 5 Years	Percent of Physicians
ANY MARKETING STRATEGY OR TECHNIQUE	40%
Studied demographic information on your community for its effects on your practice in coming years	27
Used surveys to learn about patient satisfaction with various aspects of your practice	13
Opened a satellite office or ambulatory care center	11
Advertised your practice on radio or TV or in a newspaper or magazine	9
Developed a patient newsletter	8
Employed an advertising, public relations or marketing firm or consultant	4
Developed a written marketing plan for your practice	4
Located practice in a "non-traditional" setting, such as a shopping center or store front	1

*Percents are accurate within ± 2%.

Table 3

USE OF MARKETING STRATEGIES AND TECHNIQUES IN THE LAST 5 YEARS
BY PHYSICIAN CHARACTERISTIC

Physician Characteristic	Percent of Physicians Employing any Marketing Strategies or Techniques*
Years of Practice	
10 or less	46
More than 10	38
Type of Practice	
Solo	32
Group and other	53
Region	
Northeast	39
North Central	41
South	35
West	48
Major Specialty Group	
General and Family Practice	33
Medical	51
Surgical	38
Other	38

*The strategies and techniques considered are the same as those in Table 2. Percents are accurate within ± 3%.

As shown in Table 3, the extent to which physicians have adopted marketing approaches varies by physician characteristic. Similar to their stronger response in changing their services, physicians in practice 10 years or less are more likely than older physicians to have adopted new marketing approaches in the last five years in response to competition.

While only 32% of physicians in solo practice have employed some marketing strategy, 53% of those in group and other types of practice have employed some marketing in the last five years. This suggests that many of the marketing approaches considered may be more cost-effective in non-solo practices because of the ability to spread costs over larger numbers of physicians.

Differences in the extent of marketing responses to competition were also found by region and specialty group. In the West, 48% of physicians adopted marketing responses in contrast to 40% of physicians in all regions combined. This is probably explained by greater competitive pressures in the West due to a higher physician-population ratio than in the rest of the country. By specialty, 51% of medical specialists have used marketing strategies and techniques in the last 5 years compared to only 38% of surgical and other specialists and 33% of general and family practitioners. The reason for these differences by specialty is not directly apparent.

DETAILED TABULATIONS

TABLE 1. MEAN NUMBER OF WEEKS PRACTICED, 1982*

	ALL PHYSICIANS**	SPECIALTY								
		GP/FP	INT MED	SURG	PED	OB/GYN	RAD	PSYCH	ANES	PATH
ALL PHYSICIANS	46.7	46.9	46.7	46.5	47.1	47.2	46.1	47.2	45.8	47.5
CENSUS DIVISION										
NEW ENGLAND	46.1	43.3	47.5	44.8	47.5	46.4	46.1	47.0	43.4	48.8
MIDDLE ATLANTIC	46.9	47.9	45.7	46.4	46.7	46.9	47.2	47.4	47.2	47.0
EAST NORTH CENTRAL	46.7	46.3	47.1	47.4	46.6	47.7	45.3	46.9	45.5	47.4
WEST NORTH CENTRAL	46.2	46.5	45.7	46.7	47.9	45.1	45.3	45.8	44.8	47.0
SOUTH ATLANTIC	47.0	47.4	46.7	47.5	47.3	46.6	46.3	47.5	47.6	48.1
EAST SOUTH CENTRAL	47.7	47.2	48.9	47.1	48.5	47.9	48.4	48.5	47.7	
WEST SOUTH CENTRAL	46.8	48.1	48.7	45.5	47.5	46.7	45.4	47.1	44.8	46.4
MOUNTAIN	46.3	46.7	46.2	45.8	.	47.2	43.2	47.2	46.9	
PACIFIC	46.4	46.9	45.8	45.8	46.1	48.7	46.2	47.5	44.8	47.5
TYPE OF PRACTICE										
SOLO	47.1	47.0	47.6	47.0	47.6	47.4	48.1	47.1	46.0	49.6
NON-SOLO	46.4	46.8	46.1	46.0	46.8	47.0	45.8	47.4	45.8	47.3
LOCATION										
NONMETROPOLITAN	46.6	46.8	46.6	46.3	46.8	47.5	46.0	47.1	45.8	47.9
METROPOLITAN										
LESS THAN 1,000,000	46.8	47.2	47.1	46.6	47.4	46.5	45.6	47.3	46.0	47.1
1,000,000 AND OVER	46.9	46.6	46.4	47.1	47.0	48.5	47.7	47.5	45.3	48.2
EMPLOYMENT STATUS										
SELF-EMPLOYED	47.0	47.3	47.5	46.9	47.2	47.4	46.2	46.9	45.8	48.0
EMPLOYEE	45.7	45.2	44.6	44.1	46.8	45.7	45.7	48.0	46.0	47.0
PHYSICIAN AGE										
LESS THAN 36 YEARS	44.5	46.0	44.0	43.0	45.4	42.9	44.5	43.7	45.5	44.3
36-45 YEARS	47.0	47.7	47.4	46.3	47.3	48.0	46.1	47.8	45.8	47.1
46-55 YEARS	47.4	47.6	47.8	47.4	47.6	47.2	46.9	47.9	46.4	48.1
56-65 YEARS	47.1	46.9	47.4	47.4	47.7	47.9	45.8	47.0	46.6	48.8
66 OR MORE YEARS	46.4	46.0	47.7	46.1	46.6	46.8	46.0	47.0	46.6	.

SOURCE: 1983 AMA SOCIOECONOMIC MONITORING SYSTEM CORE SURVEY.

*SEE APPENDIX FOR INFORMATION ON DEFINITIONS AND COMPUTATION PROCEDURES.
**INCLUDES PHYSICIANS IN SPECIALTIES NOT LISTED SEPARATELY.
. INDICATES FEWER THAN TEN OBSERVATIONS.

TABLE 1 (CONTINUED). STANDARD ERROR OF THE MEAN NUMBER OF WEEKS PRACTICED, 1982*

	ALL PHYSICIANS**	SPECIALTY								
		GP/FP	INT MED	SURG	PED	OB/GYN	RAD	PSYCH	ANES	PATH
ALL PHYSICIANS	0.10	0.31	0.27	0.22	0.35	0.33	0.27	0.23	0.39	0.39
CENSUS DIVISION										
NEW ENGLAND	0.43	2.71	0.59	1.37	0.56	0.68	0.50	0.38	2.75	0.59
MIDDLE ATLANTIC	0.23	0.70	0.80	0.57	0.64	1.09	0.40	0.40	0.52	1.06
EAST NORTH CENTRAL	0.23	0.82	0.54	0.25	0.90	0.61	0.49	0.75	0.69	1.38
WEST NORTH CENTRAL	0.38	0.89	1.53	0.36	1.17	1.81	0.95	1.76	1.97	0.81
SOUTH ATLANTIC	0.25	0.80	0.58	0.44	1.05	0.83	0.62	0.63	0.47	0.57
EAST SOUTH CENTRAL	0.27	0.75	0.32	0.59	0.52	0.61	0.84	0.31	0.68	
WEST SOUTH CENTRAL	0.37	0.82	0.47	0.89	1.25	1.74	1.67	1.22	1.49	1.59
MOUNTAIN	0.44	1.03	1.43	0.95	.	0.68	2.10	0.49	1.05	
PACIFIC	0.28	0.73	0.90	0.63	1.07	0.27	0.67	0.37	1.25	0.41
TYPE OF PRACTICE										
SOLO	0.16	0.42	0.36	0.29	0.68	0.58	1.29	0.28	0.91	0.45
NON-SOLO	0.13	0.45	0.39	0.33	0.40	0.33	0.26	0.39	0.41	0.43
LOCATION										
NONMETROPOLITAN	0.15	0.39	0.40	0.35	0.59	0.37	0.36	0.30	0.65	0.46
METROPOLITAN										
LESS THAN 1,000,000	0.16	0.54	0.39	0.30	0.49	0.68	0.52	0.47	0.53	0.69
1,000,000 AND OVER	0.28	1.13	0.81	0.53	0.48	0.44	0.48	0.49	1.24	0.74
EMPLOYMENT STATUS										
SELF-EMPLOYED	0.10	0.31	0.26	0.20	0.44	0.29	0.27	0.30	0.47	0.27
EMPLOYEE	0.27	0.96	0.73	1.01	0.57	1.56	0.67	0.25	0.67	0.77
PHYSICIAN AGE										
LESS THAN 36 YEARS	0.42	0.95	0.91	1.40	1.41	2.58	1.34	1.71	0.89	2.40
36-45 YEARS	0.16	0.50	0.46	0.39	0.50	0.25	0.36	0.33	0.61	0.78
46-55 YEARS	0.14	0.59	0.29	0.20	0.48	0.70	0.37	0.18	0.86	0.31
56-65 YEARS	0.18	0.63	0.34	0.24	0.50	0.34	0.66	0.41	0.56	0.41
66 OR MORE YEARS	0.36	0.78	0.43	0.87	0.75	0.92	1.56	0.61		

SOURCE: 1983 AMA SOCIOECONOMIC MONITORING SYSTEM CORE SURVEY.

*SEE APPENDIX FOR INFORMATION ON DEFINITIONS AND COMPUTATION PROCEDURES.
**INCLUDES PHYSICIANS IN SPECIALTIES NOT LISTED SEPARATELY.
. INDICATES FEWER THAN TEN OBSERVATIONS.

TABLE 2. MEAN NUMBER OF WEEKS PRACTICED PER YEAR, 1973-75, 1977-79, 1981-82*

	1973	1974	1975	1977	1978	1979	1981**	1982**
ALL PHYSICIANS	47.2	47.2	47.2	47.0	47.4	46.9	46.6	46.7
SPECIALTY								
GENERAL/FAMILY PRACTICE	47.4	47.5	47.4	47.2	47.8	47.3	47.2	46.9
INTERNAL MEDICINE	47.1	47.3	47.2	47.1	47.2	46.7	46.2	46.7
SURGERY	46.9	47.2	46.9	47.0	47.0	46.7	46.6	46.5
PEDIATRICS	47.5	47.6	47.3	47.2	48.2	46.8	46.8	47.1
OBSTETRICS/GYNECOLOGY	47.7	47.4	47.3	47.4	47.9	47.5	46.6	47.2
RADIOLOGY	47.1	46.7	47.4	47.2	46.8	46.5	46.1	46.1
PSYCHIATRY	47.4	47.4	47.4	46.9	47.7	47.0	47.1	47.2
ANESTHESIOLOGY	46.9	46.5	46.2	45.9	45.8	46.5	46.0	45.8
CENSUS DIVISION								
NEW ENGLAND	46.6	47.3	47.2	46.4	46.8	46.5	46.3	46.1
MIDDLE ATLANTIC	46.7	47.1	47.0	47.0	47.3	46.7	46.5	46.9
EAST NORTH CENTRAL	47.1	46.9	46.4	46.4	47.1	46.4	46.3	46.7
WEST NORTH CENTRAL	47.2	47.2	47.5	47.1	47.4	47.3	46.1	46.2
SOUTH ATLANTIC	47.9	47.6	47.6	47.4	47.8	47.5	47.2	47.0
EAST SOUTH CENTRAL	48.1	47.5	47.1	47.7	47.9	47.5	47.3	47.7
WEST SOUTH CENTRAL	47.9	47.9	47.4	47.6	48.0	47.4	47.2	46.8
MOUNTAIN	47.2	47.2	47.3	46.7	47.3	47.2	46.5	46.3
PACIFIC	47.1	47.0	47.4	47.0	47.2	46.5	46.0	46.4
TYPE OF PRACTICE								
SOLO	47.4	47.4	47.3	47.2	47.7	47.3	46.9	47.1
NON-SOLO	46.9	47.0	47.0	46.7	47.1	46.5	46.3	46.4
LOCATION								
NONMETROPOLITAN	47.5	47.3	47.2	46.9	47.7	47.4	46.6	46.6
METROPOLITAN								
LESS THAN 1,000,000	47.3	47.3	47.2	47.0	47.4	47.1	46.7	46.8
1,000,000 AND OVER	47.1	47.1	47.1	47.0	47.4	46.6	46.0	46.9
PHYSICIAN AGE								
LESS THAN 36 YEARS	46.3	46.2	46.7	43.9	44.4	44.8	43.9	44.5
36-45 YEARS	47.5	47.5	47.4	47.8	47.5	47.2	47.0	47.0
46-55 YEARS	47.6	47.5	47.4	48.0	48.0	47.4	47.1	47.4
56-65 YEARS	47.2	47.3	47.2	47.1	47.8	47.2	47.1	47.1
66 OR MORE YEARS	46.4	46.7	46.2	46.2	47.2	46.8	46.7	46.4

SOURCE: 1981-82, AMA SOCIOECONOMIC MONITORING SYSTEM CORE SURVEYS; 1973-79, AMA PERIODIC SURVEYS OF PHYSICIANS.

*DATA, OTHER THAN IN THE SPECIALTY BREAKDOWN, ARE BASED ON RESPONSES FROM PHYSICIANS IN ALL SPECIALTIES. SEE APPENDIX FOR INFORMATION ON DEFINITIONS AND COMPUTATION PROCEDURES.

**CAUTION SHOULD BE OBSERVED IN COMPARING 1981 AND 1982 RESULTS WITH RESULTS FOR PREVIOUS YEARS BECAUSE OF CHANGES IN METHODOLOGY MADE IN THE TRANSITION FROM THE PERIODIC SURVEYS OF PHYSICIANS.

TABLE 2 (CONTINUED). STANDARD ERROR OF THE MEAN NUMBER OF WEEKS PRACTICED PER YEAR, 1973-79, 1981, 1982**

	1973	1974	1975	1977	1978	1979	1981**	1982**
ALL PHYSICIANS	0.06	0.06	0.07	0.09	0.08	0.09	0.10	0.10
SPECIALTY								
GENERAL/FAMILY PRACTICE	0.14	0.15	0.15	0.21	0.16	0.21	0.25	0.31
INTERNAL MEDICINE	0.16	0.15	0.18	0.22	0.19	0.22	0.31	0.27
SURGERY	0.13	0.12	0.13	0.18	0.16	0.18	0.21	0.22
PEDIATRICS	0.22	0.20	0.30	0.34	0.22	0.40	0.39	0.35
OBSTETRICS/GYNECOLOGY	0.22	0.22	0.24	0.29	0.27	0.23	0.45	0.33
RADIOLOGY	0.21	0.28	0.20	0.36	0.41	0.41	0.25	0.27
PSYCHIATRY	0.19	0.23	0.19	0.32	0.23	0.29	0.27	0.23
ANESTHESIOLOGY	0.21	0.25	0.31	0.48	0.44	0.32	0.32	0.39
CENSUS DIVISION								
NEW ENGLAND	0.29	0.21	0.22	0.36	0.31	0.36	0.37	0.43
MIDDLE ATLANTIC	0.14	0.13	0.16	0.19	0.15	0.20	0.25	0.23
EAST NORTH CENTRAL	0.15	0.15	0.18	0.21	0.19	0.22	0.26	0.23
WEST NORTH CENTRAL	0.23	0.24	0.21	0.36	0.28	0.28	0.42	0.38
SOUTH ATLANTIC	0.12	0.18	0.17	0.23	0.20	0.18	0.21	0.25
EAST SOUTH CENTRAL	0.26	0.37	0.37	0.41	0.36	0.42	0.45	0.27
WEST SOUTH CENTRAL	0.19	0.21	0.29	0.28	0.28	0.31	0.35	0.37
MOUNTAIN	0.26	0.32	0.27	0.51	0.34	0.38	0.34	0.44
PACIFIC	0.16	0.17	0.15	0.20	0.17	0.22	0.30	0.28
TYPE OF PRACTICE								
SOLO	0.08	0.09	0.10	0.12	0.10	0.12	0.16	0.16
NON-SOLO	0.09	0.09	0.09	0.14	0.11	0.13	0.13	0.13
LOCATION								
NONMETROPOLITAN	0.18	0.20	0.23	0.32	0.23	0.29	0.14	0.15
METROPOLITAN								
LESS THAN 1,000,000	0.09	0.10	0.11	0.14	0.13	0.13	0.16	0.16
1,000,000 AND OVER	0.09	0.09	0.10	0.12	0.10	0.13	0.36	0.28
PHYSICIAN AGE								
LESS THAN 36 YEARS	0.40	0.32	0.31	0.40	0.50	0.35	0.49	0.42
36-45 YEARS	0.11	0.09	0.11	0.11	0.13	0.15	0.15	0.16
46-55 YEARS	0.09	0.11	0.11	0.10	0.10	0.14	0.16	0.14
56-65 YEARS	0.11	0.13	0.14	0.20	0.13	0.17	0.17	0.18
66 OR MORE YEARS	0.23	0.22	0.28	0.33	0.21	0.24	0.32	0.36

SOURCE: 1981-82, AMA SOCIOECONOMIC MONITORING SYSTEM CORE SURVEYS; 1973-79, AMA PERIODIC SURVEYS OF PHYSICIANS.

*DATA, OTHER THAN IN THE SPECIALTY BREAKDOWN, ARE BASED ON RESPONSES FROM PHYSICIANS IN ALL SPECIALTIES. SEE APPENDIX FOR INFORMATION ON DEFINITIONS AND COMPUTATION PROCEDURES.

**CAUTION SHOULD BE OBSERVED IN COMPARING 1981 AND 1982 RESULTS WITH RESULTS FOR PREVIOUS YEARS BECAUSE OF CHANGES IN METHODOLOGY MADE IN THE TRANSITION FROM THE PERIODIC SURVEYS OF PHYSICIANS TO THE SOCIOECONOMIC MONITORING SYSTEM.

TABLE 3. MEAN NUMBER OF HOURS IN PROFESSIONAL ACTIVITIES PER WEEK, 1982*

| | ALL PHYSICIANS** | SPECIALTY | | | | | | | | |
		GP/FP	INT MED	SURG	PED	OB/GYN	RAD	PSYCH	ANES	PATH
ALL PHYSICIANS	56.8	57.4	58.9	57.0	57.2	58.4	59.2	50.2	59.5	51.6
CENSUS DIVISION										
NEW ENGLAND	56.4	56.6	61.3	56.8	59.6	58.5	55.9	46.4	64.7	48.3
MIDDLE ATLANTIC	55.6	54.0	56.8	55.8	56.1	59.0	57.3	53.6	61.5	52.4
EAST NORTH CENTRAL	56.7	57.8	58.2	57.4	55.2	57.6	61.9	51.0	55.1	50.8
WEST NORTH CENTRAL	58.9	59.8	58.8	61.0	60.7	61.8	63.0	50.4	59.9	50.9
SOUTH ATLANTIC	57.9	56.1	61.3	57.6	55.8	59.4	61.4	53.0	62.3	51.7
EAST SOUTH CENTRAL	58.6	61.3	62.0	56.8	56.7	57.4	61.9	46.9	61.6	57.8
WEST SOUTH CENTRAL	58.1	60.4	59.2	58.4	62.8	57.7	58.6	51.9	61.4	43.6
MOUNTAIN	56.8	56.2	59.6	59.1	59.9	57.6	54.5	42.2	57.6	56.3
PACIFIC	54.7	55.5	57.5	54.5	56.8	57.3	55.9	46.3	57.0	55.1
TYPE OF PRACTICE										
SOLO	56.3	57.3	60.0	56.1	57.5	57.8	56.9	50.7	55.5	50.0
NON-SOLO	57.2	57.5	57.9	57.9	57.1	58.9	59.4	49.4	61.5	51.9
LOCATION										
NONMETROPOLITAN	57.1	58.1	58.3	58.0	57.5	59.5	58.8	50.0	59.2	50.5
METROPOLITAN										
LESS THAN 1,000,000	56.9	56.3	60.4	56.9	57.2	57.0	59.5	50.0	60.6	52.9
1,000,000 AND OVER	55.2	56.5	57.7	52.7	56.4	58.4	60.3	51.4	57.4	49.7
EMPLOYMENT STATUS										
SELF-EMPLOYED	57.6	58.0	60.3	57.3	58.6	58.8	60.1	51.0	58.4	51.8
EMPLOYEE	55.0	55.0	55.8	56.2	54.6	57.1	58.1	48.6	61.6	51.6
PHYSICIAN AGE										
LESS THAN 36 YEARS	58.6	60.0	60.8	56.6	59.3	60.0	63.3	48.4	61.1	50.9
36-45 YEARS	58.4	59.6	60.2	58.8	56.7	60.5	63.0	51.3	61.1	51.5
46-55 YEARS	57.2	60.4	60.1	57.2	58.8	57.4	56.5	52.8	57.3	51.9
56-65 YEARS	55.8	56.7	56.3	56.8	57.8	59.9	54.2	49.0	59.5	51.1
66 OR MORE YEARS	49.4	50.4	50.3	49.6	48.2	50.5	49.0	42.6	54.3	54.4

SOURCE: 1ST-4TH QUARTER 1982 SOCIOECONOMIC MONITORING SYSTEM SURVEYS.

*SEE APPENDIX FOR INFORMATION ON DEFINITIONS AND COMPUTATION PROCEDURES.
**INCLUDES PHYSICIANS IN SPECIALTIES NOT LISTED SEPARATELY.

TABLE 3 (CONTINUED). STANDARD ERROR OF THE MEAN NUMBER OF HOURS IN PROFESSIONAL ACTIVITIES PER WEEK, 1982*

	ALL PHYSICIANS**	SPECIALTY								
		GP/FP	INT MED	SURG	PED	OB/GYN	RAD	PSYCH	ANES	PATH
ALL PHYSICIANS	0.21	0.53	0.53	0.43	0.70	0.81	0.97	0.66	0.96	1.20
CENSUS DIVISION										
NEW ENGLAND	0.83	2.58	2.23	1.98	2.22	3.24	1.92	1.53	3.32	2.66
MIDDLE ATLANTIC	0.53	1.53	1.13	1.09	1.69	2.34	2.26	1.66	2.47	3.39
EAST NORTH CENTRAL	0.54	1.33	1.34	1.07	1.56	2.50	3.11	1.52	2.29	1.72
WEST NORTH CENTRAL	0.78	1.39	1.89	1.57	4.17	2.19	5.53	3.58	4.48	1.80
SOUTH ATLANTIC	0.52	1.30	1.41	1.04	1.49	1.81	1.88	1.67	2.15	3.21
EAST SOUTH CENTRAL	0.91	2.05	2.02	1.63	2.15	3.11	4.08	3.43	7.48	7.67
WEST SOUTH CENTRAL	0.67	1.47	1.77	1.33	2.69	1.96	3.13	2.12	2.99	2.86
MOUNTAIN	0.92	2.31	2.27	2.24	2.44	2.76	3.50	3.87	2.74	5.92
PACIFIC	0.52	1.34	1.34	1.01	1.91	1.95	2.15	1.35	2.14	4.54
TYPE OF PRACTICE										
SOLO	0.33	0.72	0.86	0.68	1.11	1.24	2.73	0.84	1.73	3.15
NON-SOLO	0.28	0.76	0.65	0.55	0.91	1.06	1.04	1.07	1.13	1.30
LOCATION										
NONMETROPOLITAN	0.29	0.65	0.72	0.59	0.99	1.21	1.24	0.87	1.46	1.78
METROPOLITAN										
LESS THAN 1,000,000	0.36	0.95	0.95	0.72	1.04	1.04	1.66	1.17	1.52	1.83
1,000,000 AND OVER	0.67	2.43	1.38	1.27	2.30	2.92	4.01	1.95	2.24	3.43
EMPLOYMENT STATUS										
SELF-EMPLOYED	0.26	0.58	0.66	0.50	0.92	0.89	1.51	0.81	1.19	1.74
EMPLOYEE	0.37	1.26	0.84	0.85	1.01	1.90	1.18	1.13	1.63	1.58
PHYSICIAN AGE										
LESS THAN 36 YEARS	0.61	1.41	1.26	1.37	2.20	2.33	3.25	1.47	2.75	5.27
36-45 YEARS	0.36	1.11	0.85	0.71	1.03	1.43	1.62	1.06	1.47	1.76
46-55 YEARS	0.41	1.14	1.10	0.76	1.31	1.54	1.58	1.27	1.96	1.75
56-65 YEARS	0.48	0.97	1.28	1.03	1.63	1.73	2.04	1.62	2.31	3.60
66 OR MORE YEARS	0.73	1.29	1.91	1.71	3.13	2.60	3.30	1.93	3.11	7.70

SOURCE: 1ST-4TH QUARTER 1982 SOCIOECONOMIC MONITORING SYSTEM SURVEYS.

*SEE APPENDIX FOR INFORMATION ON DEFINITIONS AND COMPUTATION PROCEDURES.
**INCLUDES PHYSICIANS IN SPECIALTIES NOT LISTED SEPARATELY.

TABLE 4. MEAN NUMBER OF HOURS IN PATIENT CARE ACTIVITIES PER WEEK, 1982*

SPECIALTY

	ALL PHYSICIANS**	GP/FP	INT MED	SURG	PED	OB/GYN	RAD	PSYCH	ANES	PATH
ALL PHYSICIANS	51.0	53.4	52.7	51.4	51.3	53.5	54.0	43.2	54.5	40.9
CENSUS DIVISION										
NEW ENGLAND	49.7	52.5	53.9	51.6	53.0	53.1	48.5	37.9	58.2	36.1
MIDDLE ATLANTIC	49.5	49.8	50.3	49.6	49.9	53.7	53.3	45.8	56.6	42.0
EAST NORTH CENTRAL	50.8	53.9	51.9	51.9	48.9	52.9	56.6	43.2	50.0	40.1
WEST NORTH CENTRAL	53.2	56.0	51.0	55.0	55.4	56.2	57.8	43.2	53.3	44.3
SOUTH ATLANTIC	52.2	51.9	54.8	52.2	50.0	54.6	56.4	47.4	56.1	39.1
EAST SOUTH CENTRAL	53.5	57.8	56.7	51.6	51.1	52.3	54.9	43.3	58.1	46.5
WEST SOUTH CENTRAL	53.5	56.7	54.4	53.2	58.5	54.1	55.7	45.7	56.8	36.2
MOUNTAIN	51.3	52.4	53.1	54.5	54.5	54.5	50.4	35.7	54.0	41.3
PACIFIC	48.7	51.3	52.0	48.2	50.3	51.8	49.1	39.5	53.0	43.8
TYPE OF PRACTICE										
SOLO	51.1	53.5	54.4	50.7	52.4	52.9	50.5	44.1	51.5	42.5
NON-SOLO	51.0	53.3	51.3	52.0	50.7	54.1	54.3	41.9	55.9	40.6
LOCATION										
NONMETROPOLITAN	51.4	54.3	52.2	52.3	51.7	54.2	53.5	43.1	53.9	40.2
METROPOLITAN										
LESS THAN 1,000,000	51.2	52.0	54.3	51.6	51.8	52.8	54.5	43.8	55.8	41.6
1,000,000 AND OVER	48.8	52.5	50.8	46.8	48.8	53.0	54.5	42.6	52.2	39.8
EMPLOYMENT STATUS										
SELF-EMPLOYED	52.5	54.1	54.8	52.0	53.8	54.1	55.1	44.6	54.2	42.3
EMPLOYEE	47.8	50.5	48.1	49.4	46.5	51.6	52.6	40.5	54.9	40.2
PHYSICIAN AGE										
LESS THAN 36 YEARS	52.4	55.5	53.8	50.8	52.3	55.6	56.3	40.6	55.5	42.8
36-45 YEARS	52.3	54.9	54.0	52.9	50.6	55.7	57.6	44.2	55.2	42.6
46-55 YEARS	51.3	56.2	54.0	51.4	52.7	51.9	51.6	45.4	52.7	40.1
56-65 YEARS	50.5	53.1	50.4	51.7	53.3	54.8	49.8	42.4	55.2	36.5
66 OR MORE YEARS	45.1	47.5	45.6	44.5	42.7	46.2	45.6	36.1	50.0	45.3

SOURCE: 1ST-4TH QUARTER 1982 SOCIOECONOMIC MONITORING SYSTEM SURVEYS.

*SEE APPENDIX FOR INFORMATION ON DEFINITIONS AND COMPUTATION PROCEDURES.
**INCLUDES PHYSICIANS IN SPECIALTIES NOT LISTED SEPARATELY.

TABLE 4 (CONTINUED). STANDARD ERROR OF THE MEAN NUMBER OF HOURS IN PATIENT CARE ACTIVITIES PER WEEK, 1982*

	ALL PHYSICIANS**	SPECIALTY								
		GP/FP	INT MED	SURG	PED	OB/GYN	RAD	PSYCH	ANES	PATH
ALL PHYSICIANS	• 0.21	0.51	0.53	0.42	0.72	0.80	0.93	0.65	0.96	1.12
CENSUS DIVISION										
NEW ENGLAND	0.87	2.56	2.30	1.98	2.18	3.28	2.40	1.71	3.78	2.67
MIDDLE ATLANTIC	0.52	1.41	1.08	1.08	1.69	2.28	2.15	1.59	2.48	3.25
EAST NORTH CENTRAL	0.54	1.32	1.30	1.01	1.60	2.32	2.87	1.57	2.26	1.77
WEST NORTH CENTRAL	0.78	1.39	2.01	1.44	4.02	2.25	5.84	3.14	3.88	1.78
SOUTH ATLANTIC	0.52	1.26	1.42	1.02	1.63	1.88	1.81	1.65	1.86	2.84
EAST SOUTH CENTRAL	0.90	1.96	2.01	1.57	2.34	3.04	3.74	3.71	7.86	8.09
WEST SOUTH CENTRAL	0.66	1.41	1.70	1.28	2.55	1.80	3.22	1.85	3.25	2.26
MOUNTAIN	0.95	2.36	2.27	2.29	2.51	2.46	3.53	3.89	3.11	3.85
PACIFIC	0.50	1.26	1.36	0.87	2.03	1.94	1.82	1.34	2.16	3.50
TYPE OF PRACTICE										
SOLO	0.32	0.70	0.83	0.64	1.05	1.20	2.07	0.80	1.70	3.30
NON-SOLO	0.28	0.74	0.66	0.54	0.97	1.07	1.01	1.11	1.14	1.18
LOCATION										
NONMETROPOLITAN	0.28	0.62	0.73	0.55	1.02	1.18	1.16	0.84	1.42	1.33
METROPOLITAN										
LESS THAN 1,000,000	0.36	0.94	0.92	0.71	1.08	1.06	1.64	1.27	1.52	1.88
1,000,000 AND OVER	0.66	2.40	1.34	1.22	2.27	2.86	3.76	1.79	2.43	3.17
EMPLOYMENT STATUS										
SELF-EMPLOYED	0.25	0.56	0.63	0.48	0.89	0.86	1.43	0.78	1.19	1.63
EMPLOYEE	0.38	1.24	0.88	0.83	1.15	1.94	1.15	1.14	1.63	1.47
PHYSICIAN AGE										
LESS THAN 36 YEARS	0.62	1.39	1.25	1.33	2.21	2.23	2.73	1.61	2.72	5.96
36-45 YEARS	0.36	1.07	0.84	0.69	1.13	1.43	1.57	1.10	1.43	1.63
46-55 YEARS	0.41	1.12	1.08	0.74	1.33	1.56	1.52	1.24	2.03	1.50
56-65 YEARS	0.48	0.94	1.34	0.99	1.58	1.68	2.09	1.51	2.23	3.06
66 OR MORE YEARS	0.70	1.27	1.84	1.53	2.88	2.54	3.09	2.01	4.80	6.47

SOURCE: 1ST-4TH QUARTER 1982 SOCIOECONOMIC MONITORING SYSTEM SURVEYS.

*SEE APPENDIX FOR INFORMATION ON DEFINITIONS AND COMPUTATION PROCEDURES.
**INCLUDES PHYSICIANS IN SPECIALTIES NOT LISTED SEPARATELY.

TABLE 5. MEAN NUMBER OF HOURS IN PATIENT CARE ACTIVITIES PER WEEK, 1973-76, 1978-80, 1982*

	1973	1974	1975	1976	1978	1979	1980	1982**
ALL PHYSICIANS	46.1	44.5	47.5	46.5	45.4	44.9	44.5	51.0
SPECIALTY								
GENERAL/FAMILY PRACTICE	47.6	45.5	49.0	46.5	45.8	45.0	44.5	53.4
INTERNAL MEDICINE	47.5	46.2	49.2	49.3	47.8	47.2	47.4	52.7
SURGERY	47.8	46.3	48.9	47.9	48.2	46.9	46.5	51.4
PEDIATRICS	44.5	44.2	46.1	44.9	44.5	43.5	43.8	51.3
OBSTETRICS/GYNECOLOGY	48.8	48.1	51.6	49.4	47.3	47.8	45.9	53.5
RADIOLOGY	41.8	41.4	41.9	44.5	43.9	43.7	41.7	54.0
PSYCHIATRY	40.3	37.3	41.0	41.3	38.2	39.6	38.8	43.2
ANESTHESIOLOGY	48.0	44.7	47.2	47.2	46.6	44.5	46.5	54.5
CENSUS DIVISION								
NEW ENGLAND	45.5	44.3	46.5	45.7	44.2	43.4	42.9	49.7
MIDDLE ATLANTIC	43.2	41.8	45.5	45.4	43.5	43.9	42.8	49.5
EAST NORTH CENTRAL	46.4	44.8	47.7	45.9	45.6	43.9	44.1	50.8
WEST NORTH CENTRAL	49.4	45.6	49.9	48.3	47.3	46.8	48.4	53.2
SOUTH ATLANTIC	46.8	45.9	48.2	47.8	45.6	46.4	45.1	52.2
EAST SOUTH CENTRAL	50.9	48.5	52.8	49.5	49.3	47.6	48.6	53.5
WEST SOUTH CENTRAL	49.5	47.2	49.9	49.4	46.9	46.4	45.8	53.5
MOUNTAIN	47.4	46.5	48.2	46.4	49.1	46.8	46.7	51.3
PACIFIC	44.8	43.0	45.7	44.6	44.2	43.3	43.1	48.7
TYPE OF PRACTICE								
SOLO	44.7	43.3	47.1	45.7	44.2	44.8	43.9	51.1
NON-SOLO	48.1	46.1	47.9	47.2	47.3	45.0	45.2	51.0
LOCATION								
NONMETROPOLITAN	50.9	47.9	50.0	48.7	48.4	48.4	48.2	51.4
METROPOLITAN								
LESS THAN 1,000,000	47.4	45.5	48.8	47.8	47.1	46.0	45.5	51.2
1,000,000 AND OVER	44.0	42.9	45.7	44.8	43.4	43.2	43.1	48.8
PHYSICIAN AGE								
LESS THAN 36 YEARS	46.7	44.6	47.7	48.0	46.6	46.9	46.7	52.4
36-45 YEARS	48.3	45.8	48.7	48.2	47.4	46.8	46.1	52.3
46-55 YEARS	48.2	47.1	49.8	48.2	47.2	46.6	45.7	51.3
56-65 YEARS	44.4	44.1	46.1	45.6	44.2	44.4	43.7	50.5
66 OR MORE YEARS	36.5	36.2	40.2	37.3	35.2	37.4	36.4	45.1

SOURCE: 1982, AMA SOCIOECONOMIC MONITORING SYSTEM CORE SURVEYS; 1973-80, AMA PERIODIC SURVEYS OF PHYSICIANS.

*DATA, OTHER THAN IN THE SPECIALTY BREAKDOWN, INCLUDE RESPONSES FROM PHYSICIANS IN ALL SPECIALTIES. SEE APPENDIX FOR INFORMATION ON DEFINITIONS AND COMPUTATION PROCEDURES.

**CAUTION SHOULD BE OBSERVED. IN COMPARING 1982 RESULTS WITH RESULTS FOR PREVIOUS YEARS BECAUSE OF CHANGES IN METHODOLOGY MADE IN THE TRANSITION FROM THE PERIODIC SURVEYS OF PHYSICIANS TO THE SOCIOECONOMIC MONITORING SYSTEM.

TABLE 5 (CONTINUED). STANDARD ERROR OF THE MEAN NUMBER OF HOURS IN PATIENT CARE ACTIVITIES PER WEEK, 1973-76, 1978-80, 1982*

	1973	1974	1975	1976	1978	1979	1980	1982**
ALL PHYSICIANS	0.23	0.21	0.20	0.21	0.22	0.22	0.21	0.21
SPECIALTY								
GENERAL/FAMILY PRACTICE	0.53	0.44	0.43	0.45	0.48	0.51	0.47	0.51
INTERNAL MEDICINE	0.56	0.50	0.46	0.50	0.55	0.53	0.48	0.53
SURGERY	0.47	0.42	0.40	0.41	0.47	0.48	0.45	0.42
PEDIATRICS	0.79	0.84	0.70	0.74	0.77	0.76	0.77	0.72
OBSTETRICS/GYNECOLOGY	0.89	0.78	0.77	0.90	0.85	0.90	0.82	0.80
RADIOLOGY	0.78	0.73	0.77	0.65	0.62	0.74	0.76	0.93
PSYCHIATRY	0.75	0.67	0.65	0.67	0.78	0.72	0.67	0.65
ANESTHESIOLOGY	0.98	0.85	0.83	0.87	0.99	1.07	0.86	0.96
CENSUS DIVISION								
NEW ENGLAND	0.87	0.80	0.82	0.86	0.85	0.81	0.82	0.87
MIDDLE ATLANTIC	0.53	0.48	0.46	0.50	0.59	0.57	0.47	0.52
EAST NORTH CENTRAL	0.54	0.49	0.47	0.48	0.54	0.56	0.53	0.54
WEST NORTH CENTRAL	0.79	0.78	0.79	0.79	0.80	0.84	0.77	0.78
SOUTH ATLANTIC	0.66	0.55	0.52	0.55	0.54	0.59	0.50	0.52
EAST SOUTH CENTRAL	1.16	1.07	1.04	0.94	1.05	0.90	1.01	0.90
WEST SOUTH CENTRAL	0.82	0.77	0.72	0.69	0.77	0.78	0.73	0.66
MOUNTAIN	1.16	1.03	0.98	0.88	0.98	0.92	1.05	0.95
PACIFIC	0.50	0.44	0.44	0.45	0.48	0.48	0.46	0.50
TYPE OF PRACTICE								
SOLO	0.32	0.28	0.29	0.30	0.31	0.33	0.30	0.32
NON-SOLO	0.33	0.30	0.27	0.28	0.31	0.30	0.29	0.28
LOCATION								
NONMETROPOLITAN	0.73	0.64	0.56	0.62	0.68	0.69	0.72	0.28
METROPOLITAN								
LESS THAN 1,000,000	0.36	0.33	0.32	0.32	0.35	0.35	0.33	0.36
1,000,000 AND OVER	0.32	0.29	0.29	0.29	0.31	0.32	0.29	0.66
PHYSICIAN AGE								
LESS THAN 36 YEARS	0.88	0.90	0.60	0.69	0.55	0.73	0.56	0.62
36-45 YEARS	0.40	0.37	0.34	0.36	0.40	0.42	0.39	0.36
46-55 YEARS	0.39	0.36	0.35	0.36	0.39	0.39	0.39	0.41
56-65 YEARS	0.49	0.42	0.44	0.43	0.51	0.45	0.43	0.48
66 OR MORE YEARS	0.78	0.62	0.70	0.65	0.78	0.63	0.66	0.70

SOURCE: 1982, AMA SOCIOECONOMIC MONITORING SYSTEM CORE SURVEYS; 1973-80, AMA PERIODIC SURVEYS OF PHYSICIANS.

*DATA, OTHER THAN IN THE SPECIALTY BREAKDOWN, INCLUDE RESPONSES FROM PHYSICIANS IN ALL SPECIALTIES. SEE APPENDIX FOR INFORMATION ON DEFINITIONS AND COMPUTATION PROCEDURES.

**CAUTION SHOULD BE OBSERVED IN COMPARING 1982 RESULTS WITH RESULTS FOR PREVIOUS YEARS BECAUSE OF CHANGES IN METHODOLOGY MADE IN THE TRANSITION FROM THE PERIODIC SURVEYS OF PHYSICIANS TO THE SOCIOECONOMIC MONITORING SYSTEM.

TABLE 6. MEAN NUMBER OF HOURS IN DIRECT PATIENT CARE ACTIVITIES PER WEEK, 1982*

| | ALL PHYSICIANS** | SPECIALTY | | | | |
		GENERAL & FAMILY PRACTICE	INTERNAL MEDICINE	SURGERY	PEDIATRICS	OBSTETRICS/ GYNECOLOGY
ALL PHYSICIANS	47.7	49.5	47.4	48.1	45.5	49.5
CENSUS DIVISION						
NEW ENGLAND	47.2	48.2	47.2	47.6	45.5	49.3
MIDDLE ATLANTIC	45.3	45.5	45.7	46.0	44.0	48.7
EAST NORTH CENTRAL	47.6	50.4	47.2	48.3	42.6	48.7
WEST NORTH CENTRAL	50.1	52.2	46.1	52.0	49.7	52.2
SOUTH ATLANTIC	48.5	48.2	49.0	49.1	44.4	50.7
EAST SOUTH CENTRAL	50.2	54.4	51.5	48.3	46.3	49.3
WEST SOUTH CENTRAL	50.1	52.6	48.7	49.7	51.0	51.2
MOUNTAIN	48.8	49.1	46.2	51.7	49.8	50.2
PACIFIC	45.7	46.7	47.1	45.2	45.6	47.6
TYPE OF PRACTICE						
SOLO	48.0	49.3	49.3	47.5	46.4	48.5
NON-SOLO	47.5	49.8	45.9	48.6	44.9	50.4
LOCATION						
NONMETROPOLITAN	48.4	50.4	47.0	48.9	45.4	50.3
METROPOLITAN						
LESS THAN 1,000,000	47.8	48.1	48.8	48.5	46.6	48.9
1,000,000 AND OVER	44.6	48.2	46.0	42.8	42.8	48.3
EMPLOYMENT STATUS						
SELF-EMPLOYED	49.0	50.0	49.4	48.6	47.8	50.1
EMPLOYEE	44.3	47.5	43.1	46.1	41.0	47.5
PHYSICIAN AGE						
LESS THAN 36 YEARS	48.8	51.7	48.7	46.9	46.4	51.8
36-45 YEARS	48.7	50.8	48.4	49.7	45.2	51.9
46-55 YEARS	48.5	52.0	48.8	48.1	47.0	47.7
56-65 YEARS	47.5	49.5	45.1	48.6	47.0	50.6
66 OR MORE YEARS	41.8	43.7	41.3	41.1	35.2	42.4

SOURCE: 1ST-4TH QUARTER 1982 AMA SOCIOECONOMIC MONITORING SYSTEM SURVEYS.

*SEE APPENDIX FOR INFORMATION ON DEFINITIONS AND COMPUTATION PROCEDURES.
**EXCLUDES RADIOLOGY, PSYCHIATRY, ANESTHESIOLOGY AND PATHOLOGY, BUT OTHERWISE INCLUDES SPECIALTIES NOT LISTED SEPARATELY.

TABLE 6 (CONTINUED). STANDARD ERROR OF THE MEAN NUMBER OF HOURS IN DIRECT PATIENT CARE ACTIVITIES PER WEEK, 1982*

	ALL PHYSICIANS**	SPECIALTY				
		GENERAL & FAMILY PRACTICE	INTERNAL MEDICINE	SURGERY	PEDIATRICS	OBSTETRICS/ GYNECOLOGY
ALL PHYSICIANS	0.22	0.49	0.50	0.40	0.66	0.77
CENSUS DIVISION						
NEW ENGLAND	0.96	2.30	2.11	1.80	2.29	3.26
MIDDLE ATLANTIC	0.55	1.32	1.03	1.04	1.56	2.25
EAST NORTH CENTRAL	0.57	1.27	1.23	0.98	1.35	2.10
WEST NORTH CENTRAL	0.76	1.29	2.00	1.35	3.25	2.67
SOUTH ATLANTIC	0.57	1.20	1.37	0.96	1.55	1.80
EAST SOUTH CENTRAL	0.88	1.86	1.85	1.53	2.14	2.88
WEST SOUTH CENTRAL	0.68	1.35	1.63	1.21	2.06	1.74
MOUNTAIN	1.04	2.26	2.36	2.14	2.35	2.52
PACIFIC	0.54	1.19	1.27	0.84	1.98	1.83
TYPE OF PRACTICE						
SOLO	0.34	0.67	0.78	0.61	0.97	1.14
NON-SOLO	0.30	0.71	0.64	0.52	0.87	1.03
LOCATION						
NONMETROPOLITAN	0.30	0.60	0.70	0.53	0.94	1.14
METROPOLITAN						
LESS THAN 1,000,000	0.38	0.89	0.87	0.68	1.00	1.05
1,000,000 AND OVER	0.69	2.28	1.23	1.17	1.98	2.65
EMPLOYMENT STATUS						
SELF-EMPLOYED	0.26	0.53	0.59	0.46	0.79	0.83
EMPLOYEE	0.43	1.19	0.87	0.80	1.07	1.86
PHYSICIAN AGE						
LESS THAN 36 YEARS	0.65	1.31	1.21	1.30	2.05	2.20
36-45 YEARS	0.38	1.02	0.83	0.64	1.02	1.31
46-55 YEARS	0.44	1.08	0.97	0.70	1.22	1.48
56-65 YEARS	0.49	0.89	1.22	0.94	1.38	1.62
66 OR MORE YEARS	0.74	1.23	1.78	1.51	2.47	2.63

SOURCE: 1ST-4TH QUARTER 1982 AMA SOCIOECONOMIC MONITORING SYSTEM SURVEYS.

*SEE APPENDIX FOR INFORMATION ON DEFINITIONS AND COMPUTATION PROCEDURES.
**EXCLUDES RADIOLOGY, PSYCHIATRY, ANESTHESIOLOGY AND PATHOLOGY, BUT OTHERWISE INCLUDES SPECIALTIES NOT LISTED SEPARATELY.

TABLE 7. MEAN NUMBER OF OFFICE HOURS PER WEEK, 1982*

	ALL PHYSICIANS**	SPECIALTY				
		GENERAL & FAMILY PRACTICE	INTERNAL MEDICINE	SURGERY	PEDIATRICS	OBSTETRICS/ GYNECOLOGY
ALL PHYSICIANS	26.4	33.1	26.2	22.1	32.1	26.9
CENSUS DIVISION						
NEW ENGLAND	25.8	30.6	27.2	22.0	36.1	25.0
MIDDLE ATLANTIC	24.3	30.0	24.9	19.7	32.2	23.1
EAST NORTH CENTRAL	24.9	32.0	25.3	20.7	28.6	25.0
WEST NORTH CENTRAL	26.6	33.0	24.6	20.7	31.8	28.2
SOUTH ATLANTIC	27.1	33.9	26.7	23.8	31.0	28.1
EAST SOUTH CENTRAL	28.2	35.3	25.6	21.8	33.5	28.7
WEST SOUTH CENTRAL	28.7	35.1	27.3	23.7	36.5	29.4
MOUNTAIN	26.5	35.2	25.3	23.2	31.9	28.0
PACIFIC	27.5	33.1	28.5	23.2	32.5	28.5
TYPE OF PRACTICE						
SOLO	28.3	33.6	28.6	23.2	33.6	27.1
NON-SOLO	24.8	32.5	24.3	21.0	31.2	26.8
LOCATION						
NONMETROPOLITAN	26.9	33.6	26.7	21.9	32.3	27.6
METROPOLITAN						
LESS THAN 1,000,000	26.2	32.7	25.9	22.7	32.2	26.8
1,000,000 AND OVER	25.1	30.6	25.5	20.9	31.1	24.8
EMPLOYMENT STATUS						
SELF-EMPLOYED	28.0	33.6	28.1	23.0	35.6	27.8
EMPLOYEE	22.2	31.0	22.2	18.8	25.5	24.0
PHYSICIAN AGE						
LESS THAN 36 YEARS	24.8	33.8	23.1	20.9	31.4	25.9
36-45 YEARS	24.9	33.6	25.2	21.3	29.9	27.3
46-55 YEARS	27.4	34.2	29.6	22.3	35.3	26.1
56-65 YEARS	28.5	33.5	27.4	22.8	35.8	28.1
66 OR MORE YEARS	27.3	30.2	27.8	23.9	26.7	26.5

SOURCE: 1ST-4TH QUARTER 1982 AMA SOCIOECONOMIC MONITORING SYSTEM SURVEYS.

*SEE APPENDIX FOR INFORMATION ON DEFINITIONS AND COMPUTATION PROCEDURES.
**EXCLUDES RADIOLOGY, PSYCHIATRY, ANESTHESIOLOGY AND PATHOLOGY, BUT OTHERWISE INCLUDES SPECIALTIES NOT LISTED SEPARATELY.

TABLE 7 (CONTINUED). STANDARD ERROR OF THE MEAN NUMBER OF OFFICE HOURS PER WEEK, 1982*

			SPECIALTY			
	ALL PHYSICIANS**	GENERAL & FAMILY PRACTICE	INTERNAL MEDICINE	SURGERY	PEDIATRICS	OBSTETRICS/ GYNECOLOGY
ALL PHYSICIANS	0.20	0.33	0.41	0.32	0.64	0.44
CENSUS DIVISION						
NEW ENGLAND	0.84	1.70	1.51	1.28	2.26	1.49
MIDDLE ATLANTIC	0.48	1.05	0.92	0.81	1.36	1.15
EAST NORTH CENTRAL	0.49	0.79	1.09	0.78	1.45	0.98
WEST NORTH CENTRAL	0.75	0.90	1.79	1.27	2.73	1.57
SOUTH ATLANTIC	0.49	0.81	1.03	0.79	1.84	1.02
EAST SOUTH CENTRAL	0.75	1.04	1.70	1.19	1.99	1.59
WEST SOUTH CENTRAL	0.60	0.87	1.47	0.97	1.79	0.87
MOUNTAIN	0.97	1.53	2.11	1.63	2.92	2.05
PACIFIC	0.45	0.80	0.89	0.67	1.81	1.30
TYPE OF PRACTICE						
SOLO	0.27	0.44	0.59	0.45	0.83	0.64
NON-SOLO	0.28	0.48	0.57	0.44	0.90	0.61
LOCATION						
NONMETROPOLITAN	0.27	0.41	0.57	0.43	0.93	0.64
METROPOLITAN						
LESS THAN 1,000,000	0.34	0.58	0.77	0.53	0.98	0.66
1,000,000 AND OVER	0.54	1.41	0.93	0.95	1.90	1.37
EMPLOYMENT STATUS						
SELF-EMPLOYED	0.21	0.35	0.44	0.35	0.62	0.45
EMPLOYEE	0.41	0.84	0.85	0.66	1.25	1.10
PHYSICIAN AGE						
LESS THAN 36 YEARS	0.57	0.79	1.00	1.04	1.64	1.24
36-45 YEARS	0.35	0.69	0.67	0.52	1.11	0.70
46-55 YEARS	0.40	0.74	0.84	0.60	1.22	0.98
56-65 YEARS	0.41	0.61	1.04	0.75	1.27	0.94
66 OR MORE YEARS	0.55	0.84	1.21	1.09	2.31	1.45

SOURCE: 1ST-4TH QUARTER 1982 AMA SOCIOECONOMIC MONITORING SYSTEM SURVEYS.

*SEE APPENDIX FOR INFORMATION ON DEFINITIONS AND COMPUTATION PROCEDURES.
**EXCLUDES RADIOLOGY, PSYCHIATRY, ANESTHESIOLOGY AND PATHOLOGY, BUT OTHERWISE INCLUDES SPECIALTIES NOT LISTED SEPARATELY.

TABLE 8. MEAN NUMBER OF OFFICE HOURS PER WEEK, 1973-76, 1978-80, 1982*

	1973	1974	1975	1976	1978	1979	1980	1982**
ALL PHYSICIANS	29.3	28.8	29.5	29.8	31.0	28.4	28.2	26.4
SPECIALTY								
GENERAL/FAMILY PRACTICE	34.4	33.2	34.4	34.9	36.0	33.5	33.8	33.1
INTERNAL MEDICINE	29.5	29.0	30.1	29.9	30.9	28.1	27.9	26.2
SURGERY	22.7	22.5	22.8	23.7	25.3	22.7	22.4	22.1
PEDIATRICS	36.2	35.7	35.5	36.0	37.4	34.9	35.1	32.1
OBSTETRICS/GYNECOLOGY	27.6	28.4	28.3	28.7	30.7	29.3	29.0	26.9
CENSUS DIVISION								
NEW ENGLAND	27.7	26.8	27.7	27.6	29.1	26.3	27.2	25.8
MIDDLE ATLANTIC	26.2	27.4	27.7	27.4	28.6	26.6	25.8	24.3
EAST NORTH CENTRAL	29.0	27.0	28.3	28.7	29.4	26.4	27.0	24.9
WEST NORTH CENTRAL	29.7	27.6	29.1	29.9	30.2	28.3	28.4	26.6
SOUTH ATLANTIC	31.0	31.2	30.3	31.5	32.5	29.8	28.8	27.1
EAST SOUTH CENTRAL	31.2	31.4	33.0	30.8	33.6	29.6	29.7	28.2
WEST SOUTH CENTRAL	31.7	31.2	31.5	31.8	32.6	30.3	31.3	28.7
MOUNTAIN	31.9	29.8	29.3	30.2	32.0	28.8	28.9	26.5
PACIFIC	30.1	29.4	30.5	31.6	32.9	29.9	29.0	27.5
TYPE OF PRACTICE								
SOLO	29.2	29.0	29.7	30.3	30.9	29.0	28.8	28.3
NON-SOLO	29.5	28.5	29.2	29.3	31.0	27.7	27.5	24.8
LOCATION								
NONMETROPOLITAN	33.4	31.5	32.3	33.4	33.8	31.3	31.2	26.9
METROPOLITAN								
LESS THAN 1,000,000	29.4	28.8	29.6	29.8	31.3	28.4	28.5	26.2
1,000,000 AND OVER	28.2	28.1	28.5	29.1	30.0	27.6	27.2	25.1
PHYSICIAN AGE								
LESS THAN 36 YEARS	28.0	28.4	30.7	30.0	29.8	29.3	28.4	24.8
36-45 YEARS	29.4	27.8	28.3	29.4	30.1	27.4	27.1	24.9
46-55 YEARS	30.3	30.4	30.8	30.8	32.9	28.9	28.8	27.4
56-65 YEARS	29.5	29.5	29.6	30.3	31.6	29.1	29.1	28.5
66 OR MORE YEARS	26.8	26.5	28.0	27.7	28.5	27.5	27.2	27.3

SOURCE: 1982, AMA SOCIOECONOMIC MONITORING SYSTEM CORE SURVEYS; 1973-80, AMA PERIODIC SURVEYS OF PHYSICIANS.

*DATA ARE BASED ON INFORMATION FROM PHYSICIANS IN ALL SPECIALTIES EXCLUDING PSYCHIATRY, RADIOLOGY, ANESTHESIOLOGY AND PATHOLOGY. RESULTS FOR YEARS PRIOR TO 1982, OTHER THAN IN THE SPECIALTY BREAKDOWN, MAY DIFFER FROM PREVIOUSLY REPORTED RESULTS BECAUSE OF THE SPECIALTY EXCLUSIONS. SEE APPENDIX FOR INFORMATION ON DEFINITIONS AND COMPUTATION PROCEDURES.
**CAUTION SHOULD BE OBSERVED IN COMPARING 1982 RESULTS WITH RESULTS FOR PREVIOUS YEARS BECAUSE OF CHANGES IN METHODOLOGY MADE IN THE TRANSITION FROM THE PERIODIC SURVEYS OF PHYSICIANS TO THE SOCIOECONOMIC MONITORING SYSTEM.

TABLE 8 (CONTINUED). STANDARD ERROR OF THE MEAN NUMBER OF OFFICE HOURS PER WEEK, 1973-76, 1978-80, 1982*

	1973	1974	1975	1976	1978	1979	1980	1982**
ALL PHYSICIANS	0.21	0.20	0.19	0.20	0.24	0.21	0.19	0.20
SPECIALTY								
GENERAL/FAMILY PRACTICE	0.36	0.34	0.32	0.36	0.42	0.38	0.33	0.33
INTERNAL MEDICINE	0.44	0.41	0.36	0.41	0.52	0.40	0.38	0.41
SURGERY	0.36	0.34	0.31	0.34	0.46	0.37	0.34	0.32
PEDIATRICS	0.61	0.72	0.62	0.65	0.84	0.67	0.65	0.64
OBSTETRICS/GYNECOLOGY	0.54	0.48	0.46	0.55	0.66	0.53	0.48	0.44
CENSUS DIVISION								
NEW ENGLAND	0.88	0.83	0.72	0.78	0.94	0.88	0.80	0.84
MIDDLE ATLANTIC	0.46	0.45	0.45	0.46	0.63	0.50	0.48	0.48
EAST NORTH CENTRAL	0.45	0.46	0.44	0.47	0.57	0.48	0.46	0.49
WEST NORTH CENTRAL	0.76	0.69	0.67	0.72	0.85	0.78	0.67	0.75
SOUTH ATLANTIC	0.59	0.55	0.52	0.56	0.62	0.53	0.48	0.49
EAST SOUTH CENTRAL	0.96	1.05	0.90	0.98	1.25	0.85	0.97	0.75
WEST SOUTH CENTRAL	0.77	0.67	0.65	0.71	0.81	0.72	0.67	0.60
MOUNTAIN	1.07	0.98	0.84	0.83	1.07	0.86	0.88	0.97
PACIFIC	0.47	0.43	0.41	0.46	0.51	0.47	0.43	0.45
TYPE OF PRACTICE								
SOLO	0.27	0.26	0.26	0.27	0.31	0.28	0.25	0.27
NON-SOLO	0.32	0.30	0.27	0.30	0.38	0.31	0.29	0.28
LOCATION								
NONMETROPOLITAN	0.58	0.54	0.46	0.56	0.67	0.57	0.55	0.27
METROPOLITAN								
LESS THAN 1,000,000	0.33	0.31	0.29	0.31	0.39	0.32	0.30	0.34
1,000,000 AND OVER	0.30	0.29	0.28	0.29	0.34	0.30	0.28	0.54
PHYSICIAN AGE								
LESS THAN 36 YEARS	0.77	0.91	0.66	0.78	0.68	0.74	0.57	0.57
36-45 YEARS	0.38	0.38	0.34	0.38	0.46	0.41	0.38	0.35
46-55 YEARS	0.40	0.37	0.34	0.39	0.44	0.40	0.38	0.40
56-65 YEARS	0.42	0.39	0.39	0.39	0.54	0.42	0.40	0.41
66 OR MORE YEARS	0.59	0.51	0.54	0.51	0.74	0.50	0.51	0.55

SOURCE: 1982, AMA SOCIOECONOMIC MONITORING SYSTEM CORE SURVEYS; 1973-80, AMA PERIODIC SURVEYS OF PHYSICIANS.

*DATA ARE BASED ON INFORMATION FROM PHYSICIANS IN ALL SPECIALTIES EXCLUDING PSYCHIATRY, RADIOLOGY, ANESTHESIOLOGY AND PATHOLOGY. RESULTS FOR YEARS PRIOR TO 1982, OTHER THAN IN THE SPECIALTY BREAKDOWN, MAY DIFFER FROM PREVIOUSLY REPORTED RESULTS BECAUSE OF THE SPECIALTY EXCLUSIONS. SEE APPENDIX FOR INFORMATION ON DEFINITIONS AND COMPUTATION PROCEDURES.
**CAUTION SHOULD BE OBSERVED IN COMPARING 1982 RESULTS WITH RESULTS FOR PREVIOUS YEARS BECAUSE OF CHANGES IN METHODOLOGY MADE IN THE TRANSITION FROM THE PERIODIC SURVEYS OF PHYSICIANS TO THE SOCIOECONOMIC MONITORING SYSTEM.

TABLE 9. MEAN NUMBER OF HOURS ON HOSPITAL ROUNDS PER WEEK, 1982*

	ALL PHYSICIANS**	SPECIALTY				
		GENERAL & FAMILY PRACTICE	INTERNAL MEDICINE	SURGERY	PEDIATRICS	OBSTETRICS/ GYNECOLOGY
ALL PHYSICIANS	9.4	8.4	15.2	9.6	8.5	6.4
CENSUS DIVISION						
NEW ENGLAND	8.7	8.3	14.7	8.7	6.3	5.0
MIDDLE ATLANTIC	9.5	8.0	14.6	9.9	7.6	5.8
EAST NORTH CENTRAL	10.6	10.2	15.9	10.5	10.1	7.1
WEST NORTH CENTRAL	10.7	9.3	14.8	12.4	12.2	6.6
SOUTH ATLANTIC	9.6	7.9	16.7	9.6	7.7	7.0
EAST SOUTH CENTRAL	10.3	9.6	18.8	10.0	8.8	6.6
WEST SOUTH CENTRAL	9.9	9.6	16.7	9.4	8.8	6.1
MOUNTAIN	8.7	6.3	16.6	8.8	11.9	7.2
PACIFIC	7.4	6.0	11.7	7.8	7.3	5.8
TYPE OF PRACTICE						
SOLO	9.5	8.1	14.8	9.5	8.7	6.6
NON-SOLO	9.4	8.8	15.6	9.7	8.4	6.1
LOCATION						
NONMETROPOLITAN	9.3	8.5	14.4	9.6	8.1	6.6
METROPOLITAN						
LESS THAN 1,000,000	9.7	8.1	16.9	9.7	9.6	6.3
1,000,000 AND OVER	9.4	8.7	14.4	8.9	7.4	5.6
EMPLOYMENT STATUS						
SELF-EMPLOYED	9.7	8.6	15.8	9.6	8.4	6.6
EMPLOYEE	8.7	7.5	13.9	9.4	8.7	5.5
PHYSICIAN AGE						
LESS THAN 36 YEARS	10.5	9.1	17.4	10.0	9.5	5.9
36-45 YEARS	10.1	8.5	17.5	9.9	8.8	6.7
46-55 YEARS	9.3	8.9	14.0	9.4	8.9	5.9
56-65 YEARS	9.0	8.4	12.6	10.2	7.7	7.1
66 OR MORE YEARS	7.1	7.4	8.8	7.4	5.2	5.5

SOURCE: 1ST-4TH QUARTER 1982 AMA SOCIOECONOMIC MONITORING SYSTEM SURVEYS.

*SEE APPENDIX FOR INFORMATION ON DEFINITIONS AND COMPUTATION PROCEDURES.
**EXCLUDES RADIOLOGY, PSYCHIATRY, ANESTHESIOLOGY AND PATHOLOGY, BUT OTHERWISE INCLUDES SPECIALTIES NOT LISTED SEPARATELY.

TABLE 9 (CONTINUED). STANDARD ERROR OF THE MEAN NUMBER OF HOURS ON HOSPITAL ROUNDS PER WEEK, 1982*

	ALL PHYSICIANS**	SPECIALTY				
		GENERAL & FAMILY PRACTICE	INTERNAL MEDICINE	SURGERY	PEDIATRICS	OBSTETRICS/ GYNECOLOGY
ALL PHYSICIANS	0.13	0.22	0.38	0.21	0.33	0.22
CENSUS DIVISION						
NEW ENGLAND	0.52	1.16	1.33	0.82	0.72	0.72
MIDDLE ATLANTIC	0.33	0.68	0.85	0.51	0.60	0.54
EAST NORTH CENTRAL	0.34	0.56	0.93	0.54	1.10	0.64
WEST NORTH CENTRAL	0.49	0.58	1.32	1.09	2.04	0.71
SOUTH ATLANTIC	0.35	0.58	0.96	0.59	0.74	0.61
EAST SOUTH CENTRAL	0.47	0.81	1.25	0.73	0.78	0.79
WEST SOUTH CENTRAL	0.41	0.64	1.34	0.61	0.84	0.63
MOUNTAIN	0.55	0.66	1.68	0.93	1.41	0.94
PACIFIC	0.29	0.40	0.96	0.43	0.86	0.49
TYPE OF PRACTICE						
SOLO	0.19	0.29	0.54	0.33	0.53	0.36
NON-SOLO	0.18	0.33	0.52	0.28	0.42	0.27
LOCATION						
NONMETROPOLITAN	0.18	0.28	0.51	0.29	0.47	0.35
METROPOLITAN						
LESS THAN 1,000,000	0.23	0.36	0.66	0.37	0.54	0.32
1,000,000 AND OVER	0.41	1.00	1.00	0.61	0.94	0.63
EMPLOYMENT STATUS						
SELF-EMPLOYED	0.15	0.24	0.46	0.25	0.36	0.26
EMPLOYEE	0.26	0.52	0.67	0.41	0.68	0.41
PHYSICIAN AGE						
LESS THAN 36 YEARS	0.41	0.56	0.89	0.86	0.90	0.46
36-45 YEARS	0.26	0.44	0.70	0.35	0.59	0.43
46-55 YEARS	0.25	0.44	0.70	0.41	0.64	0.36
56-65 YEARS	0.25	0.46	0.77	0.45	0.64	0.44
66 OR MORE YEARS	0.34	0.52	1.02	0.67	1.00	1.03

SOURCE: 1ST-4TH QUARTER 1982 AMA SOCIOECONOMIC MONITORING SYSTEM SURVEYS.

*SEE APPENDIX FOR INFORMATION ON DEFINITIONS AND COMPUTATION PROCEDURES.
**EXCLUDES RADIOLOGY, PSYCHIATRY, ANESTHESIOLOGY AND PATHOLOGY, BUT OTHERWISE INCLUDES SPECIALTIES NOT LISTED SEPARATELY.

TABLE 10. MEAN NUMBER OF HOURS ON HOSPITAL ROUNDS PER WEEK, 1973-76, 1982*

	1973	1974	1975	1976	1982**
ALL PHYSICIANS	10.5	10.1	10.6	13.3	9.4
SPECIALTY					
GENERAL/FAMILY PRACTICE	9.3	8.7	9.1	10.6	8.4
INTERNAL MEDICINE	14.7	14.6	15.3	17.0	15.2
SURGERY	11.2	10.9	11.1	15.7	9.6
PEDIATRICS	8.2	7.4	8.3	8.5	8.5
OBSTETRICS/GYNECOLOGY	8.5	7.4	8.4	12.7	6.4
CENSUS DIVISION					
NEW ENGLAND	10.7	9.9	11.1	13.7	8.7
MIDDLE ATLANTIC	10.5	9.5	10.5	14.4	9.5
EAST NORTH CENTRAL	11.2	11.4	11.5	14.7	10.6
WEST NORTH CENTRAL	12.5	11.1	12.5	14.5	10.7
SOUTH ATLANTIC	10.2	10.0	10.2	12.7	9.6
EAST SOUTH CENTRAL	12.1	11.3	11.5	15.6	10.3
WEST SOUTH CENTRAL	10.5	10.9	11.0	13.3	9.9
MOUNTAIN	10.4	9.9	10.5	12.6	8.7
PACIFIC	9.0	8.4	8.9	10.4	7.4
TYPE OF PRACTICE					
SOLO	10.0	9.7	10.2	12.9	9.5
NON-SOLO	11.3	10.5	10.9	13.8	9.4
LOCATION					
NONMETROPOLITAN	10.7	10.2	10.4	12.9	9.3
METROPOLITAN					
LESS THAN 1,000,000	11.0	10.7	11.0	13.9	9.7
1,000,000 AND OVER	10.1	9.5	10.2	12.9	9.4
PHYSICIAN AGE					
LESS THAN 36 YEARS	11.7	10.8	11.2	13.0	10.5
36-45 YEARS	11.9	11.7	11.6	14.7	10.1
46-55 YEARS	11.3	10.6	11.2	14.2	9.3
56-65 YEARS	9.2	9.3	10.2	12.4	9.0
66 OR MORE YEARS	7.1	7.0	6.8	9.7	7.1

SOURCE: 1982, AMA SOCIOECONOMIC MONITORING SYSTEM CORE SURVEYS; 1973-76, AMA PERIODIC SURVEYS OF PHYSICIANS.

*DATA ARE BASED ON INFORMATION FROM PHYSICIANS IN ALL SPECIALTIES EXCLUDING PSYCHIATRY, RADIOLOGY, ANESTHESIOLOGY AND PATHOLOGY. RESULTS FOR YEARS PRIOR TO 1982, OTHER THAN IN THE SPECIALTY BREAKDOWN, MAY DIFFER FROM PREVIOUSLY REPORTED RESULTS BECAUSE OF THE SPECIALTY EXCLUSIONS. SEE APPENDIX FOR INFORMATION ON DEFINITIONS AND COMPUTATION PROCEDURES.
**CAUTION SHOULD BE OBSERVED IN COMPARING 1982 RESULTS WITH RESULTS FOR PREVIOUS YEARS BECAUSE OF CHANGES IN METHODOLOGY MADE IN THE TRANSITION FROM THE PERIODIC SURVEYS OF PHYSICIANS TO THE SOCIOECONOMIC MONITORING SYSTEM.

TABLE 10 (CONTINUED). STANDARD ERROR OF THE MEAN NUMBER OF HOURS ON HOSPITAL ROUNDS PER WEEK, 1973-76, 1982*

	1973	1974	1975	1976	1982**
ALL PHYSICIANS	0.15	0.14	0.14	0.19	0.13
SPECIALTY					
GENERAL/FAMILY PRACTICE	0.25	0.22	0.22	0.30	0.22
INTERNAL MEDICINE	0.41	0.39	0.38	0.41	0.38
SURGERY	0.28	0.26	0.25	0.38	0.21
PEDIATRICS	0.40	0.33	0.35	0.43	0.33
OBSTETRICS/GYNECOLOGY	0.35	0.23	0.29	0.60	0.22
CENSUS DIVISION					
NEW ENGLAND	0.61	0.61	0.61	0.79	0.52
MIDDLE ATLANTIC	0.37	0.33	0.34	0.47	0.33
EAST NORTH CENTRAL	0.35	0.33	0.34	0.43	0.34
WEST NORTH CENTRAL	0.52	0.52	0.56	0.64	0.49
SOUTH ATLANTIC	0.41	0.37	0.36	0.48	0.35
EAST SOUTH CENTRAL	0.77	0.70	0.74	1.14	0.47
WEST SOUTH CENTRAL	0.46	0.49	0.46	0.61	0.41
MOUNTAIN	0.79	0.58	0.63	0.85	0.55
PACIFIC	0.33	0.31	0.31	0.37	0.29
TYPE OF PRACTICE					
SOLO	0.20	0.19	0.19	0.25	0.19
NON-SOLO	0.23	0.21	0.20	0.28	0.18
LOCATION					
NONMETROPOLITAN	0.40	0.36	0.30	0.56	0.18
METROPOLITAN					
LESS THAN 1,000,000	0.24	0.23	0.24	0.30	0.23
1,000,000 AND OVER	0.22	0.20	0.21	0.26	0.41
PHYSICIAN AGE					
LESS THAN 36 YEARS	0.66	0.74	0.50	0.68	0.41
36-45 YEARS	0.30	0.29	0.27	0.36	0.26
46-55 YEARS	0.26	0.26	0.25	0.35	0.25
56-65 YEARS	0.29	0.25	0.30	0.38	0.25
66 OR MORE YEARS	0.41	0.32	0.33	0.43	0.34

SOURCE: 1982, AMA SOCIOECONOMIC MONITORING SYSTEM CORE SURVEYS; 1973-76, AMA PERIODIC SURVEYS OF PHYSICIANS.

*DATA ARE BASED ON INFORMATION FROM PHYSICIANS IN ALL SPECIALTIES EXCLUDING PSYCHIATRY, RADIOLOGY, ANESTHESIOLOGY AND PATHOLOGY. RESULTS FOR YEARS PRIOR TO 1982, OTHER THAN IN THE SPECIALTY BREAKDOWN, MAY DIFFER FROM PREVIOUSLY REPORTED RESULTS BECAUSE OF THE SPECIALTY EXCLUSIONS. SEE APPENDIX FOR INFORMATION ON DEFINITIONS AND COMPUTATION PROCEDURES.
**CAUTION SHOULD BE OBSERVED IN COMPARING 1982 RESULTS WITH RESULTS FOR PREVIOUS YEARS BECAUSE OF CHANGES IN METHODOLOGY MADE IN THE TRANSITION FROM THE PERIODIC SURVEYS OF PHYSICIANS TO THE SOCIOECONOMIC MONITORING SYSTEM.

TABLE 11. MEAN NUMBER OF HOURS IN SURGERY PER WEEK, 1982*

| | ALL PHYSICIANS** | SPECIALTY | | | | |
		GENERAL & FAMILY PRACTICE	INTERNAL MEDICINE	SURGERY	PEDIATRICS	OBSTETRICS/ GYNECOLOGY
ALL PHYSICIANS	6.0	2.4	0.8	13.2	0.9	14.1
CENSUS DIVISION						
NEW ENGLAND	5.8	1.3	0.5	12.1	0.3	17.2
MIDDLE ATLANTIC	5.6	0.9	0.8	13.0	0.7	16.4
EAST NORTH CENTRAL	6.3	3.2	1.3	14.2	0.3	14.8
WEST NORTH CENTRAL	6.7	4.2	1.0	15.2	0.8	14.7
SOUTH ATLANTIC	5.8	1.1	0.7	12.8	0.9	13.7
EAST SOUTH CENTRAL	5.7	1.8	0.5	13.1	0.8	12.1
WEST SOUTH CENTRAL	6.6	2.4	0.8	13.7	1.7	14.9
MOUNTAIN	6.5	3.2	0.6	15.3	1.2	13.4
PACIFIC	5.6	2.9	0.8	11.8	1.4	11.1
TYPE OF PRACTICE						
SOLO	5.5	2.2	0.6	11.8	0.8	12.4
NON-SOLO	6.5	2.7	1.0	14.6	0.9	15.6
LOCATION						
NONMETROPOLITAN	6.1	2.5	0.8	14.1	0.8	14.3
METROPOLITAN						
LESS THAN 1,000,000	6.2	2.0	0.9	13.0	1.0	13.8
1,000,000 AND OVER	5.1	3.2	0.7	10.2	0.8	14.6
EMPLOYMENT STATUS						
SELF-EMPLOYED	6.3	2.5	0.8	13.1	0.8	14.1
EMPLOYEE	5.2	2.0	0.9	13.8	0.9	14.1
PHYSICIAN AGE						
LESS THAN 36 YEARS	4.3	2.6	0.7	11.9	1.1	16.9
36-45 YEARS	7.1	2.5	1.2	15.0	1.2	15.9
46-55 YEARS	6.8	2.4	0.8	13.4	0.5	13.7
56-65 YEARS	5.8	2.6	0.6	12.8	0.4	14.3
66 OR MORE YEARS	3.5	1.9	0.1	7.9	0.3	7.2

SOURCE: 1ST-4TH QUARTER 1982 AMA SOCIOECONOMIC MONITORING SYSTEM SURVEYS.

*SEE APPENDIX FOR INFORMATION ON DEFINITIONS AND COMPUTATION PROCEDURES.
**EXCLUDES RADIOLOGY, PSYCHIATRY, ANESTHESIOLOGY AND PATHOLOGY, BUT OTHERWISE INCLUDES SPECIALTIES NOT LISTED SEPARATELY.

TABLE 11 (CONTINUED). STANDARD ERROR OF THE MEAN NUMBER OF HOURS IN SURGERY PER WEEK, 1982*

	ALL PHYSICIANS**	SPECIALTY				
		GENERAL & FAMILY PRACTICE	INTERNAL MEDICINE	SURGERY	PEDIATRICS	OBSTETRICS/ GYNECOLOGY
ALL PHYSICIANS	0.13	0.13	0.11	0.26	0.10	0.51
CENSUS DIVISION						
NEW ENGLAND	0.56	0.38	0.22	0.99	0.10	2.26
MIDDLE ATLANTIC	0.35	0.30	0.25	0.63	0.18	1.55
EAST NORTH CENTRAL	0.34	0.40	0.39	0.64	0.09	1.18
WEST NORTH CENTRAL	0.48	0.37	0.61	0.94	0.40	1.42
SOUTH ATLANTIC	0.34	0.28	0.23	0.64	0.29	1.26
EAST SOUTH CENTRAL	0.53	0.35	0.35	1.24	0.58	1.56
WEST SOUTH CENTRAL	0.42	0.35	0.30	0.71	0.73	1.55
MOUNTAIN	0.63	0.54	0.25	1.39	0.35	1.59
PACIFIC	0.28	0.30	0.23	0.55	0.26	0.93
TYPE OF PRACTICE						
SOLO	0.18	0.17	0.12	0.35	0.13	0.69
NON-SOLO	0.20	0.19	0.18	0.36	0.15	0.71
LOCATION						
NONMETROPOLITAN	0.18	0.16	0.17	0.34	0.13	0.74
METROPOLITAN						
LESS THAN 1,000,000	0.23	0.20	0.18	0.45	0.20	0.76
1,000,000 AND OVER	0.36	0.72	0.20	0.68	0.24	1.53
EMPLOYMENT STATUS						
SELF-EMPLOYED	0.16	0.15	0.14	0.29	0.09	0.56
EMPLOYEE	0.25	0.26	0.19	0.54	0.26	1.15
PHYSICIAN AGE						
LESS THAN 36 YEARS	0.31	0.31	0.20	0.86	0.28	1.30
36-45 YEARS	0.26	0.23	0.20	0.45	0.22	0.94
46-55 YEARS	0.29	0.28	0.25	0.47	0.13	0.97
56-65 YEARS	0.29	0.26	0.32	0.56	0.19	1.10
66 OR MORE YEARS	0.28	0.34	0.04	0.67	0.16	1.04

SOURCE: 1ST-4TH QUARTER 1982 AMA SOCIOECONOMIC MONITORING SYSTEM SURVEYS.

*SEE APPENDIX FOR INFORMATION ON DEFINITIONS AND COMPUTATION PROCEDURES.
**EXCLUDES RADIOLOGY, PSYCHIATRY, ANESTHESIOLOGY AND PATHOLOGY, BUT OTHERWISE INCLUDES SPECIALTIES NOT LISTED SEPARATELY.

TABLE 12. MEAN NUMBER OF TOTAL PATIENT VISITS PER WEEK, 1982*

| | | SPECIALTY | | | |
	ALL PHYSICIANS**	GENERAL & FAMILY PRACTICE	INTERNAL MEDICINE	SURGERY	PEDIATRICS	OBSTETRICS/ GYNECOLOGY
ALL PHYSICIANS	131.8	160.6	118.9	118.8	134.9	128.2
CENSUS DIVISION						
NEW ENGLAND	124.6	140.8	116.9	116.0	125.4	125.3
MIDDLE ATLANTIC	122.5	152.2	116.0	116.6	125.1	111.8
EAST NORTH CENTRAL	135.7	169.9	118.9	124.0	127.3	130.5
WEST NORTH CENTRAL	143.5	169.7	127.4	131.1	136.7	136.2
SOUTH ATLANTIC	138.0	153.5	120.8	130.8	141.8	139.6
EAST SOUTH CENTRAL	156.2	215.8	153.8	123.9	133.9	133.1
WEST SOUTH CENTRAL	145.2	175.8	125.7	129.5	164.5	149.7
MOUNTAIN	124.9	139.3	103.5	117.2	150.8	113.4
PACIFIC	112.1	130.9	107.4	93.0	130.4	114.9
TYPE OF PRACTICE						
SOLO	126.3	156.8	118.5	107.9	134.1	107.0
NON-SOLO	136.9	166.1	119.3	129.2	135.5	146.5
LOCATION						
NONMETROPOLITAN	132.7	161.9	116.2	118.0	134.6	129.2
METROPOLITAN						
LESS THAN 1,000,000	137.0	163.8	125.5	124.5	142.6	135.6
1,000,000 AND OVER	112.4	136.3	113.9	103.9	114.4	104.2
EMPLOYMENT STATUS						
SELF-EMPLOYED	135.1	163.3	123.5	118.8	143.3	128.3
EMPLOYEE	123.0	149.3	108.9	118.9	118.7	127.7
PHYSICIAN AGE						
LESS THAN 36 YEARS	123.6	145.3	112.8	101.9	126.5	132.2
36-45 YEARS	131.5	154.5	119.3	122.3	132.6	136.1
46-55 YEARS	140.1	188.3	131.4	121.3	151.6	132.7
56-65 YEARS	138.5	169.8	122.0	126.1	138.8	123.1
66 OR MORE YEARS	113.0	134.3	94.7	95.4	105.8	103.8

SOURCE: 1ST-4TH QUARTER 1982 AMA SOCIOECONOMIC MONITORING SYSTEM SURVEYS.

*SEE APPENDIX FOR INFORMATION ON DEFINITIONS AND COMPUTATION PROCEDURES.
**EXCLUDES RADIOLOGY, PSYCHIATRY, ANESTHESIOLOGY AND PATHOLOGY, BUT OTHERWISE INCLUDES SPECIALTIES NOT LISTED SEPARATELY.

TABLE 12 (CONTINUED). STANDARD ERROR OF THE MEAN NUMBER OF TOTAL PATIENT VISITS PER WEEK, 1982*

	ALL PHYSICIANS**	SPECIALTY				
		GENERAL & FAMILY PRACTICE	INTERNAL MEDICINE	SURGERY	PEDIATRICS	OBSTETRICS/ GYNECOLOGY
ALL PHYSICIANS	1.13	2.76	2.24	1.81	3.19	3.35
CENSUS DIVISION						
NEW ENGLAND	3.90	10.80	7.42	6.75	10.10	11.58
MIDDLE ATLANTIC	2.62	7.36	4.76	4.99	7.20	6.27
EAST NORTH CENTRAL	2.83	6.67	4.91	4.73	7.54	8.18
WEST NORTH CENTRAL	4.05	7.10	11.43	6.84	11.17	8.70
SOUTH ATLANTIC	3.01	6.69	5.83	5.29	8.35	10.39
EAST SOUTH CENTRAL	5.56	13.77	12.06	5.48	10.75	11.30
WEST SOUTH CENTRAL	3.73	8.89	7.94	5.26	12.33	9.75
MOUNTAIN	4.08	8.65	8.59	7.32	13.82	8.69
PACIFIC	2.30	5.27	5.22	3.16	8.78	8.62
TYPE OF PRACTICE						
SOLO	1.60	3.66	3.48	2.33	5.01	3.51
NON-SOLO	1.59	4.19	2.90	2.71	4.14	5.16
LOCATION						
NONMETROPOLITAN	1.57	3.49	3.20	2.39	4.61	5.30
METROPOLITAN						
LESS THAN 1,000,000	1.90	5.08	3.78	3.08	5.09	4.97
1,000,000 AND OVER	2.98	9.42	5.52	5.83	8.47	6.85
EMPLOYMENT STATUS						
SELF-EMPLOYED	1.31	3.03	2.74	1.96	3.85	3.95
EMPLOYEE	2.21	6.58	3.79	4.40	5.42	6.01
PHYSICIAN AGE						
LESS THAN 36 YEARS	2.63	5.85	4.61	4.63	8.04	7.58
36-45 YEARS	1.88	4.93	3.83	2.75	5.02	7.32
46-55 YEARS	2.39	6.26	4.84	3.43	6.70	5.86
56-65 YEARS	2.71	5.43	5.84	5.03	7.91	6.10
66 OR MORE YEARS	3.83	7.43	6.80	5.72	12.51	12.32

SOURCE: 1ST-4TH QUARTER 1982 AMA SOCIOECONOMIC MONITORING SYSTEM SURVEYS.

*SEE APPENDIX FOR INFORMATION ON DEFINITIONS AND COMPUTATION PROCEDURES.
**EXCLUDES RADIOLOGY, PSYCHIATRY, ANESTHESIOLOGY AND PATHOLOGY, BUT OTHERWISE INCLUDES SPECIALTIES NOT LISTED SEPARATELY.

TABLE 13. MEAN NUMBER OF TOTAL PATIENT VISITS PER WEEK, 1975-76, 1978-80, 1982*

	1975	1976	1978	1979	1980	1982**
ALL PHYSICIANS	139.2	137.2	136.3	129.6	117.0	131.8
SPECIALTY						
GENERAL/FAMILY PRACTICE	177.2	167.8	180.0	157.5	142.8	160.6
INTERNAL MEDICINE	124.7	124.3	118.6	117.4	104.7	118.9
SURGERY	119.6	122.2	110.8	115.9	99.7	118.8
PEDIATRICS	140.2	146.1	148.1	138.9	141.1	134.9
OBSTETRICS/GYNECOLOGY	131.8	133.2	126.2	125.9	113.2	128.2
CENSUS DIVISION						
NEW ENGLAND	119.9	117.4	107.6	106.5	104.2	124.6
MIDDLE ATLANTIC	124.1	125.4	123.0	122.6	109.5	122.5
EAST NORTH CENTRAL	149.0	154.3	144.3	140.1	123.3	135.7
WEST NORTH CENTRAL	165.0	154.2	152.0	144.8	133.4	143.5
SOUTH ATLANTIC	142.2	134.6	134.8	132.0	119.6	138.0
EAST SOUTH CENTRAL	193.3	178.0	189.5	166.2	149.8	156.2
WEST SOUTH CENTRAL	157.7	158.8	143.3	140.4	132.7	145.2
MOUNTAIN	130.1	126.6	134.6	129.3	114.8	124.9
PACIFIC	119.6	118.5	124.5	112.0	101.3	112.1
TYPE OF PRACTICE						
SOLO	132.8	133.7	132.7	124.3	112.2	126.3
NON-SOLO	146.4	141.0	141.3	135.4	121.9	136.9
LOCATION						
NONMETROPOLITAN	178.4	172.1	178.7	162.7	148.9	132.7
METROPOLITAN						
LESS THAN 1,000,000	147.3	145.2	141.1	136.4	121.6	137.0
1,000,000 AND OVER	119.7	121.9	118.5	115.3	106.7	112.4
PHYSICIAN AGE						
LESS THAN 36 YEARS	133.9	125.3	117.7	122.0	109.2	123.6
36-45 YEARS	143.0	145.4	135.2	130.3	120.2	131.5
46-55 YEARS	158.4	150.7	156.3	142.4	128.5	140.1
56-65 YEARS	134.1	132.6	131.9	133.8	120.0	138.5
66 OR MORE YEARS	97.5	99.6	107.0	101.8	86.5	113.0

SOURCE: 1982, AMA SOCIOECONOMIC MONITORING SYSTEM CORE SURVEYS; 1975-80, AMA PERIODIC SURVEYS OF PHYSICIANS.

*DATA ARE BASED ON INFORMATION FROM PHYSICIANS IN ALL SPECIALTIES EXCLUDING PSYCHIATRY, RADIOLOGY, ANESTHESIOLOGY AND PATHOLOGY. RESULTS FOR YEARS PRIOR TO 1982, OTHER THAN IN THE SPECIALTY BREAKDOWN, MAY DIFFER FROM PREVIOUSLY REPORTED RESULTS BECAUSE OF THE SPECIALTY EXCLUSIONS. SEE APPENDIX FOR INFORMATION ON DEFINITIONS AND COMPUTATION PROCEDURES.
**CAUTION SHOULD BE OBSERVED IN COMPARING 1982 RESULTS WITH RESULTS FOR PREVIOUS YEARS BECAUSE OF CHANGES IN METHODOLOGY MADE IN THE TRANSITION FROM THE PERIODIC SURVEYS OF PHYSICIANS TO THE SOCIOECONOMIC MONITORING SYSTEM.

TABLE 13 (CONTINUED). STANDARD ERROR OF THE MEAN NUMBER OF TOTAL PATIENT VISITS PER WEEK, 1975-76, 1978-80, 1982*

	1975	1976	1978	1979	1980	1982**
ALL PHYSICIANS	1.37	1.32	1.98	1.33	1.16	1.13
SPECIALTY						
GENERAL/FAMILY PRACTICE	3.19	3.02	4.27	3.02	2.64	2.76
INTERNAL MEDICINE	2.65	2.44	3.56	2.50	2.12	2.24
SURGERY	2.03	2.15	3.10	2.29	1.79	1.81
PEDIATRICS	4.35	4.72	6.47	3.90	3.77	3.19
OBSTETRICS/GYNECOLOGY	3.78	3.58	4.88	3.42	3.26	3.35
CENSUS DIVISION						
NEW ENGLAND	4.57	3.80	5.24	3.70	4.18	3.90
MIDDLE ATLANTIC	2.82	2.94	4.59	3.07	2.88	2.62
EAST NORTH CENTRAL	3.29	3.63	4.79	3.37	3.24	2.83
WEST NORTH CENTRAL	6.33	5.10	7.04	6.24	4.90	4.05
SOUTH ATLANTIC	3.39	3.28	5.60	3.30	2.73	3.01
EAST SOUTH CENTRAL	8.75	7.38	11.59	7.14	6.13	5.56
WEST SOUTH CENTRAL	5.58	4.80	6.83	4.95	4.38	3.73
MOUNTAIN	5.60	4.61	8.02	5.29	4.37	4.08
PACIFIC	2.64	2.57	3.64	2.49	2.02	2.30
TYPE OF PRACTICE						
SOLO	1.92	1.83	2.69	1.80	1.63	1.60
NON-SOLO	1.93	1.88	2.91	1.95	1.65	1.59
LOCATION						
NONMETROPOLITAN	4.55	4.59	6.60	4.67	4.36	1.57
METROPOLITAN						
LESS THAN 1,000,000	2.10	2.08	3.02	2.00	1.75	1.90
1,000,000 AND OVER	1.76	1.70	2.54	1.80	1.58	2.98
PHYSICIAN AGE						
LESS THAN 36 YEARS	4.50	4.23	4.64	4.25	2.56	2.63
36-45 YEARS	2.54	2.45	3.42	2.37	2.18	1.88
46-55 YEARS	2.66	2.57	3.85	2.62	2.45	2.39
56-65 YEARS	2.74	2.62	4.37	2.90	2.57	2.71
66 OR MORE YEARS	3.39	3.28	7.97	3.33	3.17	3.83

SOURCE: 1982, AMA SOCIOECONOMIC MONITORING SYSTEM CORE SURVEYS; 1975-80, AMA PERIODIC SURVEYS OF PHYSICIANS.

*DATA ARE BASED ON INFORMATION FROM PHYSICIANS IN ALL SPECIALTIES EXCLUDING PSYCHIATRY, RADIOLOGY, ANESTHESIOLOGY AND PATHOLOGY. RESULTS FOR YEARS PRIOR TO 1982, OTHER THAN IN THE SPECIALTY BREAKDOWN, MAY DIFFER FROM PREVIOUSLY REPORTED RESULTS BECAUSE OF THE SPECIALTY EXCLUSIONS. SEE APPENDIX FOR INFORMATION ON DEFINITIONS AND COMPUTATION PROCEDURES.
**CAUTION SHOULD BE OBSERVED IN COMPARING 1982 RESULTS WITH RESULTS FOR PREVIOUS YEARS BECAUSE OF CHANGES IN METHODOLOGY MADE IN THE TRANSITION FROM THE PERIODIC SURVEYS OF PHYSICIANS TO THE SOCIOECONOMIC MONITORING SYSTEM.

TABLE 14. MEAN NUMBER OF OFFICE VISITS PER WEEK, 1982*

		SPECIALTY				
	ALL PHYSICIANS**	GENERAL & FAMILY PRACTICE	INTERNAL MEDICINE	SURGERY	PEDIATRICS	OBSTETRICS/ GYNECOLOGY
ALL PHYSICIANS	81.8	115.0	61.6	69.2	100.8	93.7
CENSUS DIVISION						
NEW ENGLAND	74.6	91.3	66.2	65.8	107.7	86.1
MIDDLE ATLANTIC	73.7	106.1	61.6	63.9	95.0	78.5
EAST NORTH CENTRAL	80.4	115.3	58.8	68.2	93.8	100.2
WEST NORTH CENTRAL	87.9	120.4	67.0	66.4	97.4	93.4
SOUTH ATLANTIC	83.2	112.3	59.2	78.3	95.9	98.8
EAST SOUTH CENTRAL	98.0	153.1	63.8	71.6	101.6	96.2
WEST SOUTH CENTRAL	90.5	122.3	57.2	76.4	131.3	107.3
MOUNTAIN	78.7	108.7	57.4	70.5	100.9	87.0
PACIFIC	78.7	102.6	66.7	62.7	102.9	92.8
TYPE OF PRACTICE						
SOLO	85.0	114.2	65.7	68.8	104.8	79.8
NON-SOLO	78.9	116.1	58.3	69.6	98.3	105.7
LOCATION						
NONMETROPOLITAN	83.8	116.5	62.8	68.9	100.0	94.2
METROPOLITAN						
LESS THAN 1,000,000	82.9	116.4	58.8	73.9	107.0	98.2
1,000,000 AND OVER	69.7	95.6	63.9	55.6	87.8	79.3
EMPLOYMENT STATUS						
SELF-EMPLOYED	87.8	118.0	66.9	71.6	115.1	95.8
EMPLOYEE	65.5	102.4	50.1	60.8	73.9	86.8
PHYSICIAN AGE						
LESS THAN 36 YEARS	65.7	100.6	47.8	54.4	86.1	89.9
36-45 YEARS	76.1	108.8	58.4	68.5	94.1	101.8
46-55 YEARS	89.6	132.1	73.3	72.4	118.5	95.4
56-65 YEARS	93.8	122.8	71.0	74.5	115.6	90.8
66 OR MORE YEARS	80.6	101.8	61.4	63.3	79.8	79.6

SOURCE: 1ST-4TH QUARTER 1982 AMA SOCIOECONOMIC MONITORING SYSTEM SURVEYS.

*SEE APPENDIX FOR INFORMATION ON DEFINITIONS AND COMPUTATION PROCEDURES.
**EXCLUDES RADIOLOGY, PSYCHIATRY, ANESTHESIOLOGY AND PATHOLOGY, BUT OTHERWISE INCLUDES SPECIALTIES NOT LISTED SEPARATELY.

TABLE 14 (CONTINUED). STANDARD ERROR OF THE MEAN NUMBER OF OFFICE VISITS PER WEEK, 1982*

SPECIALTY

	ALL PHYSICIANS**	GENERAL & FAMILY PRACTICE	INTERNAL MEDICINE	SURGERY	PEDIATRICS	OBSTETRICS/ GYNECOLOGY
ALL PHYSICIANS	0.90	2.09	1.46	1.32	2.95	2.82
CENSUS DIVISION						
NEW ENGLAND	3.19	8.28	5.14	5.08	10.95	8.95
MIDDLE ATLANTIC	2.14	6.12	4.02	3.49	6.12	4.45
EAST NORTH CENTRAL	2.20	4.91	3.14	3.26	7.16	6.80
WEST NORTH CENTRAL	3.50	5.75	7.90	5.81	11.36	7.77
SOUTH ATLANTIC	2.29	5.31	3.13	3.37	7.05	9.21
EAST SOUTH CENTRAL	4.27	10.36	5.63	4.45	10.49	8.16
WEST SOUTH CENTRAL	3.01	5.89	4.66	4.37	11.72	7.87
MOUNTAIN	3.91	7.45	6.97	7.15	15.41	7.35
PACIFIC	1.94	4.14	3.33	2.61	8.12	8.46
TYPE OF PRACTICE						
SOLO	1.26	2.77	2.15	1.85	4.08	2.74
NON-SOLO	1.28	3.20	1.96	1.92	4.04	4.56
LOCATION						
NONMETROPOLITAN	1.27	2.63	2.04	1.87	4.34	4.65
METROPOLITAN						
LESS THAN 1,000,000	1.49	3.96	2.26	2.17	4.67	3.86
1,000,000 AND OVER	2.32	5.91	4.38	3.59	7.49	6.15
EMPLOYMENT STATUS						
SELF-EMPLOYED	1.03	2.24	1.75	1.46	3.22	3.39
EMPLOYEE	1.72	5.36	2.49	3.08	5.23	4.58
PHYSICIAN AGE						
LESS THAN 36 YEARS	2.07	4.42	2.88	3.55	6.69	5.79
36-45 YEARS	1.51	3.66	2.29	2.11	4.86	6.46
46-55 YEARS	1.82	4.64	3.16	2.34	6.25	4.38
56-65 YEARS	2.13	4.06	4.21	3.69	6.82	4.67
66 OR MORE YEARS	3.13	6.09	4.63	4.48	10.24	11.37

SOURCE: 1ST-4TH QUARTER 1982 AMA SOCIOECONOMIC MONITORING SYSTEM SURVEYS.

*SEE APPENDIX FOR INFORMATION ON DEFINITIONS AND COMPUTATION PROCEDURES.
**EXCLUDES RADIOLOGY, PSYCHIATRY, ANESTHESIOLOGY AND PATHOLOGY, BUT OTHERWISE INCLUDES SPECIALTIES NOT LISTED SEPARATELY.

TABLE 15. MEAN NUMBER OF OFFICE VISITS PER WEEK, 1973-76, 1978-80, 1982*

	1973	1974	1975	1976	1978	1979	1980	1982**
ALL PHYSICIANS	105.8	95.0	100.8	97.5	98.5	91.3	88.6	81.8
SPECIALTY								
GENERAL/FAMILY PRACTICE	145.5	129.0	138.5	129.6	133.2	119.8	116.3	115.0
INTERNAL MEDICINE	79.4	71.6	79.6	73.3	73.6	69.3	66.1	61.6
SURGERY	81.1	71.7	74.7	77.2	75.8	75.2	70.0	69.2
PEDIATRICS	134.9	126.7	123.9	122.7	123.6	116.4	124.8	100.8
OBSTETRICS/GYNECOLOGY	98.4	95.8	104.2	100.0	102.4	100.2	96.8	93.7
CENSUS DIVISION								
NEW ENGLAND	85.9	75.6	82.3	81.5	76.5	72.5	76.6	74.6
MIDDLE ATLANTIC	84.2	81.5	87.9	85.0	87.8	81.7	81.8	73.7
EAST NORTH CENTRAL	117.4	105.3	108.1	107.4	101.7	95.4	91.3	80.4
WEST NORTH CENTRAL	117.1	101.0	115.0	105.1	107.1	99.0	95.7	87.9
SOUTH ATLANTIC	117.7	101.4	103.5	97.2	98.2	91.8	90.1	83.2
EAST SOUTH CENTRAL	131.2	113.0	136.2	122.9	134.0	119.0	108.8	98.0
WEST SOUTH CENTRAL	116.8	105.6	111.8	112.6	103.9	97.0	104.4	90.5
MOUNTAIN	109.6	100.7	92.0	92.5	100.7	93.4	83.8	78.7
PACIFIC	98.3	87.5	93.1	92.3	97.9	88.7	81.9	78.7
TYPE OF PRACTICE								
SOLO	103.7	95.8	101.2	97.9	97.2	88.6	88.0	85.0
NON-SOLO	108.7	93.9	100.3	97.0	100.4	94.2	89.2	78.9
LOCATION								
NONMETROPOLITAN	142.0	129.3	129.6	126.0	126.7	112.4	109.6	83.8
METROPOLITAN								
LESS THAN 1,000,000	110.7	97.9	104.0	101.2	100.6	96.1	92.8	82.9
1,000,000 AND OVER	92.2	83.7	88.8	87.5	89.4	81.9	80.5	69.7
PHYSICIAN AGE								
LESS THAN 36 YEARS	92.1	76.5	94.4	86.5	88.1	78.8	77.6	65.7
36-45 YEARS	111.5	95.0	100.8	101.2	99.5	88.8	89.1	76.1
46-55 YEARS	116.5	107.5	114.6	107.2	111.3	100.0	98.4	89.6
56-65 YEARS	103.7	97.5	97.7	97.7	98.3	99.3	93.0	93.8
66 OR MORE YEARS	74.2	73.0	78.7	72.8	71.6	75.2	69.8	80.6

SOURCE: 1982, AMA SOCIOECONOMIC MONITORING SYSTEM CORE SURVEYS; 1973-80, AMA PERIODIC SURVEYS OF PHYSICIANS.

*DATA ARE BASED ON INFORMATION FROM PHYSICIANS IN ALL SPECIALTIES EXCLUDING PSYCHIATRY, RADIOLOGY, ANESTHESIOLOGY AND PATHOLOGY. RESULTS FOR YEARS PRIOR TO 1982, OTHER THAN IN THE SPECIALTY BREAKDOWN, MAY DIFFER FROM PREVIOUSLY REPORTED RESULTS BECAUSE OF THE SPECIALTY EXCLUSIONS. SEE APPENDIX FOR INFORMATION ON DEFINITIONS AND COMPUTATION PROCEDURES.
**CAUTION SHOULD BE OBSERVED IN COMPARING 1982 RESULTS WITH RESULTS FOR PREVIOUS YEARS BECAUSE OF CHANGES IN METHODOLOGY MADE IN THE TRANSITION FROM THE PERIODIC SURVEYS OF PHYSICIANS TO THE SOCIOECONOMIC MONITORING SYSTEM.

TABLE 15 (CONTINUED). STANDARD ERROR OF THE MEAN NUMBER OF OFFICE VISITS PER WEEK, 1973-76, 1978-80, 1982*

	1973	1974	1975	1976	1978	1979	1980	1982**
ALL PHYSICIANS	1.17	1.14	1.10	1.09	1.26	1.09	0.98	0.90
SPECIALTY								
GENERAL/FAMILY PRACTICE	2.45	2.37	2.49	2.37	2.74	2.30	2.06	2.09
INTERNAL MEDICINE	2.01	1.87	1.98	1.64	2.32	1.73	1.38	1.46
SURGERY	1.61	1.63	1.38	1.42	1.83	1.73	1.37	1.32
PEDIATRICS	4.02	5.25	3.79	3.91	3.99	3.48	3.47	2.95
OBSTETRICS/GYNECOLOGY	2.60	2.57	2.75	2.56	3.24	3.79	2.36	2.82
CENSUS DIVISION								
NEW ENGLAND	3.82	3.60	3.61	3.16	3.44	3.24	3.46	3.19
MIDDLE ATLANTIC	2.15	2.34	2.22	2.22	2.81	2.28	2.46	2.14
EAST NORTH CENTRAL	2.87	3.20	2.73	3.28	3.04	2.59	2.68	2.20
WEST NORTH CENTRAL	4.30	4.21	4.81	3.80	5.14	5.97	3.64	3.50
SOUTH ATLANTIC	3.68	3.20	2.80	2.79	3.38	2.48	2.34	2.29
EAST SOUTH CENTRAL	5.80	5.91	6.83	6.10	7.65	6.41	5.04	4.27
WEST SOUTH CENTRAL	4.31	4.08	4.13	4.07	4.55	3.86	3.67	3.01
MOUNTAIN	5.94	5.54	4.45	3.98	5.28	4.33	3.62	3.91
PACIFIC	2.37	2.24	2.43	2.17	2.70	2.44	1.91	1.94
TYPE OF PRACTICE								
SOLO	1.52	1.55	1.62	1.48	1.71	1.38	1.32	1.26
NON-SOLO	1.84	1.67	1.45	1.59	1.83	1.71	1.44	1.28
LOCATION								
NONMETROPOLITAN	3.66	3.69	3.47	3.55	4.54	3.16	3.07	1.27
METROPOLITAN								
LESS THAN 1,000,000	1.87	1.80	1.68	1.65	1.88	1.68	1.44	1.49
1,000,000 AND OVER	1.53	1.52	1.48	1.52	1.72	1.57	1.42	2.32
PHYSICIAN AGE								
LESS THAN 36 YEARS	4.00	4.39	3.25	3.25	3.07	3.04	2.23	2.07
36-45 YEARS	2.15	2.14	2.09	2.23	2.35	1.86	1.93	1.51
46-55 YEARS	2.27	2.23	2.15	2.09	2.35	2.04	2.03	1.82
56-65 YEARS	2.30	2.40	2.15	2.16	2.84	2.81	2.09	2.13
66 OR MORE YEARS	2.94	2.47	3.03	2.41	4.18	2.60	2.47	3.13

SOURCE: 1982, AMA SOCIOECONOMIC MONITORING SYSTEM CORE SURVEYS; 1973-80, AMA PERIODIC SURVEYS OF PHYSICIANS.

*DATA ARE BASED ON INFORMATION FROM PHYSICIANS IN ALL SPECIALTIES EXCLUDING PSYCHIATRY, RADIOLOGY, ANESTHESIOLOGY AND PATHOLOGY. RESULTS FOR YEARS PRIOR TO 1982, OTHER THAN IN THE SPECIALTY BREAKDOWN, MAY DIFFER FROM PREVIOUSLY REPORTED RESULTS BECAUSE OF THE SPECIALTY EXCLUSIONS. SEE APPENDIX FOR INFORMATION ON DEFINITIONS AND COMPUTATION PROCEDURES.

**CAUTION SHOULD BE OBSERVED IN COMPARING 1982 RESULTS WITH RESULTS FOR PREVIOUS YEARS BECAUSE OF CHANGES IN METHODOLOGY MADE IN THE TRANSITION FROM THE PERIODIC SURVEYS OF PHYSICIANS TO THE SOCIOECONOMIC MONITORING SYSTEM.

TABLE 16.   MEAN NUMBER OF VISITS ON HOSPITAL ROUNDS PER WEEK, 1982*

			SPECIALTY			
	ALL PHYSICIANS**	GENERAL & FAMILY PRACTICE	INTERNAL MEDICINE	SURGERY	PEDIATRICS	OBSTETRICS/ GYNECOLOGY
ALL PHYSICIANS	34.1	30.7	45.0	42.8	23.6	27.9
CENSUS DIVISION						
NEW ENGLAND	29.0	25.4	36.1	39.8	13.1	29.6
MIDDLE ATLANTIC	33.3	28.6	41.9	44.1	21.2	24.2
EAST NORTH CENTRAL	37.9	36.0	47.3	48.7	23.1	27.8
WEST NORTH CENTRAL	39.5	35.1	48.3	55.2	28.3	25.9
SOUTH ATLANTIC	37.2	28.0	51.0	47.1	28.2	33.9
EAST SOUTH CENTRAL	43.9	47.1	72.0	45.5	24.2	31.3
WEST SOUTH CENTRAL	41.1	39.7	56.6	47.7	25.7	35.2
MOUNTAIN	28.8	20.5	39.1	39.5	40.1	23.4
PACIFIC	20.5	15.6	27.9	25.4	18.2	19.2
TYPE OF PRACTICE						
SOLO	29.9	28.6	40.5	33.5	20.1	21.7
NON-SOLO	37.9	33.7	48.6	51.8	25.7	33.3
LOCATION						
NONMETROPOLITAN	33.4	32.3	40.8	42.1	23.1	28.2
METROPOLITAN						
LESS THAN 1,000,000	36.5	28.8	54.0	45.1	27.2	30.6
1,000,000 AND OVER	30.0	24.8	39.0	38.7	15.4	19.5
EMPLOYMENT STATUS						
SELF-EMPLOYED	34.1	31.5	45.2	40.8	21.4	27.0
EMPLOYEE	34.1	27.4	44.5	49.9	27.8	30.8
PHYSICIAN AGE						
LESS THAN 36 YEARS	34.0	29.4	48.5	39.3	30.1	33.0
36-45 YEARS	36.3	29.8	50.3	46.5	23.5	27.6
46-55 YEARS	37.5	38.7	45.6	43.1	24.7	32.2
56-65 YEARS	33.7	32.0	39.9	44.7	19.4	27.5
66 OR MORE YEARS	21.0	21.7	21.8	26.3	15.4	14.4

SOURCE: 1ST-4TH QUARTER 1982 AMA SOCIOECONOMIC MONITORING SYSTEM SURVEYS.

*SEE APPENDIX FOR INFORMATION ON DEFINITIONS AND COMPUTATION PROCEDURES.
**EXCLUDES RADIOLOGY, PSYCHIATRY, ANESTHESIOLOGY AND PATHOLOGY, BUT OTHERWISE INCLUDES SPECIALTIES NOT LISTED SEPARATELY.

TABLE 16 (CONTINUED). STANDARD ERROR OF THE MEAN NUMBER OF VISITS ON HOSPITAL ROUNDS PER WEEK, 1982*

	ALL •PHYSICIANS**	SPECIALTY				
		GENERAL & FAMILY PRACTICE	INTERNAL MEDICINE	SURGERY	PEDIATRICS	OBSTETRICS/ GYNECOLOGY
ALL PHYSICIANS	0.61	1.11	1.50	1.31	1.48	1.20
CENSUS DIVISION						
NEW ENGLAND	2.28	4.97	4.87	5.10	1.66	3.80
MIDDLE ATLANTIC	1.57	3.37	3.45	3.50	2.77	3.33
EAST NORTH CENTRAL	1.53	2.47	3.52	3.53	2.83	2.49
WEST NORTH CENTRAL	2.12	2.76	6.16	4.98	5.49	3.51
SOUTH ATLANTIC	1.76	2.78	3.86	4.03	5.35	3.58
EAST SOUTH CENTRAL	2.65	5.70	7.58	4.25	3.39	3.94
WEST SOUTH CENTRAL	2.13	4.14	6.36	3.77	3.53	3.92
MOUNTAIN	2.11	2.55	4.13	5.31	6.97	2.66
PACIFIC	0.92	1.20	2.40	1.79	4.11	1.83
TYPE OF PRACTICE						
SOLO	0.78	1.47	2.06	1.50	1.64	1.47
NON-SOLO	0.92	1.70	2.15	2.08	2.13	1.78
LOCATION						
NONMETROPOLITAN	0.81	1.52	1.98	1.71	2.13	1.65
METROPOLITAN						
LESS THAN 1,000,000	1.09	1.74	2.88	2.25	2.62	2.16
1,000,000 AND OVER	1.75	3.57	3.44	4.21	2.71	2.23
EMPLOYMENT STATUS						
SELF-EMPLOYED	0.68	1.25	1.72	1.38	1.26	1.27
EMPLOYEE	1.34	2.36	2.97	3.32	3.53	3.02
PHYSICIAN AGE						
LESS THAN 36 YEARS	1.57	2.49	3.18	4.00	5.99	3.54
36-45 YEARS	1.09	2.10	2.57	2.19	2.08	1.83
46-55 YEARS	1.36	2.87	3.27	2.61	2.77	2.98
56-65 YEARS	1.43	2.44	4.09	3.16	2.28	2.42
66 OR MORE YEARS	1.28	1.97	3.85	2.89	3.34	2.41

SOURCE: 1ST-4TH QUARTER 1982 AMA SOCIOECONOMIC MONITORING SYSTEM SURVEYS.

*SEE APPENDIX FOR INFORMATION ON DEFINITIONS AND COMPUTATION PROCEDURES.
**EXCLUDES RADIOLOGY, PSYCHIATRY, ANESTHESIOLOGY AND PATHOLOGY, BUT OTHERWISE INCLUDES SPECIALTIES NOT LISTED SEPARATELY.

TABLE 17. MEAN NUMBER OF VISITS ON HOSPITAL ROUNDS PER WEEK, 1973-76, 1982*

	1973	1974	1975	1976	1982**
ALL PHYSICIANS	38.6	30.9	32.6	35.5	34.1
SPECIALTY					
GENERAL/FAMILY PRACTICE	34.2	26.8	28.5	29.5	30.7
INTERNAL MEDICINE	45.4	39.3	40.5	44.5	45.0
SURGERY	47.2	38.8	40.8	42.1	42.8
PEDIATRICS	20.6	16.7	17.3	17.2	23.6
OBSTETRICS/GYNECOLOGY	31.2	26.6	29.0	29.0	27.9
CENSUS DIVISION					
NEW ENGLAND	33.7	27.9	30.1	31.4	29.0
MIDDLE ATLANTIC	36.0	25.9	31.1	34.8	33.3
EAST NORTH CENTRAL	41.5	35.1	35.8	40.7	37.9
WEST NORTH CENTRAL	53.3	41.5	43.4	44.2	39.5
SOUTH ATLANTIC	38.3	31.0	33.0	35.5	37.2
EAST SOUTH CENTRAL	60.5	49.6	44.1	52.1	43.9
WEST SOUTH CENTRAL	44.3	38.7	40.8	42.5	41.1
MOUNTAIN	34.0	33.0	32.9	29.0	28.8
PACIFIC	26.5	20.3	21.2	23.8	20.5
TYPE OF PRACTICE					
SOLO	32.5	25.8	26.5	30.2	29.9
NON-SOLO	47.3	37.8	39.3	41.1	37.9
LOCATION					
NONMETROPOLITAN	53.1	41.8	38.8	39.7	33.4
METROPOLITAN					
LESS THAN 1,000,000	42.0	35.3	36.4	39.5	36.5
1,000,000 AND OVER	32.0	24.4	27.1	31.0	30.0
PHYSICIAN AGE					
LESS THAN 36 YEARS	37.7	25.9	30.9	34.7	34.0
36-45 YEARS	42.6	35.9	36.4	41.0	36.3
46-55 YEARS	45.0	35.6	38.1	39.0	37.5
56-65 YEARS	33.8	29.3	30.5	31.8	33.7
66 OR MORE YEARS	19.3	16.8	15.7	20.2	21.0

SOURCE: 1982, AMA SOCIOECONOMIC MONITORING SYSTEM CORE SURVEYS; 1973-76, AMA PERIODIC SURVEYS OF PHYSICIANS.

*DATA ARE BASED ON INFORMATION FROM PHYSICIANS IN ALL SPECIALTIES EXCLUDING PSYCHIATRY, RADIOLOGY, ANESTHESIOLOGY AND PATHOLOGY. RESULTS FOR YEARS PRIOR TO 1982, OTHER THAN IN THE SPECIALTY BREAKDOWN, MAY DIFFER FROM PREVIOUSLY REPORTED RESULTS BECAUSE OF THE SPECIALTY EXCLUSIONS. SEE APPENDIX FOR INFORMATION ON DEFINITIONS AND COMPUTATION PROCEDURES.
**CAUTION SHOULD BE OBSERVED IN COMPARING 1982 RESULTS WITH RESULTS FOR PREVIOUS YEARS BECAUSE OF CHANGES IN METHODOLOGY MADE IN THE TRANSITION FROM THE PERIODIC SURVEYS OF PHYSICIANS TO THE SOCIOECONOMIC MONITORING SYSTEM.

TABLE 17 (CONTINUED). STANDARD ERROR OF THE MEAN NUMBER OF VISITS ON HOSPITAL ROUNDS PER WEEK, 1973-76, 1982*

	1973	1974	1975	1976	1982**
ALL PHYSICIANS	0.73	0.60	0.61	0.66	0.61
SPECIALTY					
GENERAL/FAMILY PRACTICE	1.22	1.01	1.05	1.04	1.11
INTERNAL MEDICINE	1.61	1.47	1.40	1.40	1.50
SURGERY	1.51	1.33	1.36	1.43	1.31
PEDIATRICS	1.32	1.24	1.07	1.11	1.48
OBSTETRICS/GYNECOLOGY	1.52	1.19	1.50	1.61	1.20
CENSUS DIVISION					
NEW ENGLAND	2.16	2.14	2.14	2.07	2.28
MIDDLE ATLANTIC	1.80	1.34	1.49	1.71	1.57
EAST NORTH CENTRAL	1.69	1.36	1.51	1.58	1.53
WEST NORTH CENTRAL	2.91	2.52	2.49	2.72	2.12
SOUTH ATLANTIC	2.06	1.72	1.68	1.78	1.76
EAST SOUTH CENTRAL	4.34	4.16	3.25	3.52	2.65
WEST SOUTH CENTRAL	2.72	2.37	2.59	2.43	2.13
MOUNTAIN	2.53	2.95	2.60	2.04	2.11
PACIFIC	1.17	0.94	0.96	1.18	0.92
TYPE OF PRACTICE					
SOLO	0.81	0.69	0.69	0.77	0.78
NON-SOLO	1.31	1.05	1.01	1.07	0.92
LOCATION					
NONMETROPOLITAN	2.44	2.20	1.72	1.98	0.81
METROPOLITAN					
LESS THAN 1,000,000	1.16	1.02	1.04	1.12	1.09
1,000,000 AND OVER	0.96	0.71	0.79	0.86	1.75
PHYSICIAN AGE					
LESS THAN 36 YEARS	2.55	2.11	1.91	2.11	1.57
36-45 YEARS	1.38	1.21	1.18	1.36	1.09
46-55 YEARS	1.41	1.22	1.24	1.28	1.36
56-65 YEARS	1.47	1.16	1.26	1.22	1.43
66 OR MORE YEARS	1.40	1.21	1.13	1.41	1.28

SOURCE: 1982, AMA SOCIOECONOMIC MONITORING SYSTEM CORE SURVEYS; 1973-76, AMA PERIODIC SURVEYS OF PHYSICIANS.

*DATA ARE BASED ON INFORMATION FROM PHYSICIANS IN ALL SPECIALTIES EXCLUDING PSYCHIATRY, RADIOLOGY, ANESTHESIOLOGY AND PATHOLOGY. RESULTS FOR YEARS PRIOR TO 1982, OTHER THAN IN THE SPECIALTY BREAKDOWN, MAY DIFFER FROM PREVIOUSLY REPORTED RESULTS BECAUSE OF THE SPECIALTY EXCLUSIONS. SEE APPENDIX FOR INFORMATION ON DEFINITIONS AND COMPUTATION PROCEDURES.
**CAUTION SHOULD BE OBSERVED IN COMPARING 1982 RESULTS WITH RESULTS FOR PREVIOUS YEARS BECAUSE OF CHANGES IN METHODOLOGY MADE IN THE TRANSITION FROM THE PERIODIC SURVEYS OF PHYSICIANS TO THE SOCIOECONOMIC MONITORING SYSTEM.

TABLE 18.   MEAN NUMBER OF SURGICAL PROCEDURES PER WEEK, 1982*

				SPECIALTY		
	ALL PHYSICIANS**	GENERAL & FAMILY PRACTICE	INTERNAL MEDICINE	SURGERY	PEDIATRICS	OBSTETRICS/ GYNECOLOGY
ALL PHYSICIANS	3.3	1.4	0.6	7.2	0.6	7.8
CENSUS DIVISION						
NEW ENGLAND	3.0	0.6	0.3	6.3	0.3	8.1
MIDDLE ATLANTIC	3.0	0.3	0.6	7.1	0.5	7.2
EAST NORTH CENTRAL	3.5	1.6	0.7	8.1	0.1	8.6
WEST NORTH CENTRAL	4.0	2.7	0.8	8.7	1.2	9.5
SOUTH ATLANTIC	3.2	0.6	0.5	6.9	0.5	7.2
EAST SOUTH CENTRAL	3.3	0.9	0.4	7.5	0.2	7.2
WEST SOUTH CENTRAL	3.9	1.4	0.7	7.5	0.9	9.5
MOUNTAIN	3.3	1.9	0.4	7.3	0.9	7.6
PACIFIC	3.1	2.1	0.5	5.9	0.9	7.0
TYPE OF PRACTICE						
SOLO	2.9	1.1	0.4	6.3	0.5	6.2
NON-SOLO	3.7	1.8	0.7	8.0	0.6	9.2
LOCATION						
NONMETROPOLITAN	3.4	1.5	0.4	7.5	0.5	8.0
METROPOLITAN						
LESS THAN 1,000,000	3.6	1.3	0.8	7.2	0.7	8.3
1,000,000 AND OVER	2.5	1.4	0.5	5.4	0.6	5.7
EMPLOYMENT STATUS						
SELF-EMPLOYED	3.5	1.4	0.5	7.1	0.6	7.7
EMPLOYEE	3.0	1.6	0.8	7.4	0.5	8.2
PHYSICIAN AGE						
LESS THAN 36 YEARS	2.5	1.9	0.6	5.9	0.6	10.2
36-45 YEARS	3.9	1.6	0.9	8.1	0.8	8.5
46-55 YEARS	3.9	1.5	0.5	7.3	0.5	8.2
56-65 YEARS	3.1	1.3	0.3	7.1	0.2	7.2
66 OR MORE YEARS	1.8	0.8	0.0	4.2	0.3	3.7

SOURCE: 1ST-4TH QUARTER 1982 AMA SOCIOECONOMIC MONITORING SYSTEM SURVEYS.

*SEE APPENDIX FOR INFORMATION ON DEFINITIONS AND COMPUTATION PROCEDURES.
**EXCLUDES RADIOLOGY, PSYCHIATRY, ANESTHESIOLOGY AND PATHOLOGY, BUT OTHERWISE INCLUDES SPECIALTIES NOT LISTED SEPARATELY.

TABLE 18 (CONTINUED). STANDARD ERROR OF THE MEAN NUMBER OF SURGICAL PROCEDURES PER WEEK, 1982*

| | ALL PHYSICIANS** | SPECIALTY | | | | |
		GENERAL & FAMILY PRACTICE	INTERNAL MEDICINE	SURGERY	PEDIATRICS	OBSTETRICS/ GYNECOLOGY
ALL PHYSICIANS	0.08	0.10	0.08	0.16	0.08	0.27
CENSUS DIVISION						
NEW ENGLAND	0.29	0.19	0.16	0.54	0.23	1.05
MIDDLE ATLANTIC	0.19	0.09	0.20	0.38	0.23	0.65
EAST NORTH CENTRAL	0.21	0.16	0.20	0.51	0.05	0.68
WEST NORTH CENTRAL	0.31	0.22	0.53	0.68	0.65	1.34
SOUTH ATLANTIC	0.18	0.18	0.22	0.37	0.17	0.58
EAST SOUTH CENTRAL	0.32	0.19	0.27	0.74	0.12	0.80
WEST SOUTH CENTRAL	0.25	0.26	0.29	0.41	0.43	1.01
MOUNTAIN	0.31	0.31	0.17	0.66	0.39	0.94
PACIFIC	0.18	0.54	0.15	0.29	0.18	0.61
TYPE OF PRACTICE						
SOLO	0.10	0.09	0.08	0.20	0.11	0.32
NON-SOLO	0.12	0.21	0.13	0.24	0.12	0.39
LOCATION						
NONMETROPOLITAN	0.10	0.09	0.10	0.22	0.11	0.40
METROPOLITAN						
LESS THAN 1,000,000	0.14	0.29	0.17	0.27	0.15	0.42
1,000,000 AND OVER	0.18	0.27	0.17	0.38	0.22	0.56
EMPLOYMENT STATUS						
SELF-EMPLOYED	0.09	0.08	0.08	0.17	0.10	0.29
EMPLOYEE	0.16	0.42	0.19	0.38	0.15	0.61
PHYSICIAN AGE						
LESS THAN 36 YEARS	0.20	0.57	0.15	0.41	0.23	0.76
36-45 YEARS	0.15	0.15	0.18	0.30	0.16	0.53
46-55 YEARS	0.17	0.19	0.14	0.28	0.19	0.53
56-65 YEARS	0.15	0.13	0.14	0.33	0.07	0.42
66 OR MORE YEARS	0.15	0.16	0.02	0.36	0.17	0.58

SOURCE: 1ST-4TH QUARTER 1982 AMA SOCIOECONOMIC MONITORING SYSTEM SURVEYS.

*SEE APPENDIX FOR INFORMATION ON DEFINITIONS AND COMPUTATION PROCEDURES.
**EXCLUDES RADIOLOGY, PSYCHIATRY, ANESTHESIOLOGY AND PATHOLOGY, BUT OTHERWISE INCLUDES SPECIALTIES NOT LISTED SEPARATELY.

TABLE 19. MEAN PATIENT CARE ACTIVITIES PER WEEK: PSYCHIATRY, 1982*

	SESSIONS WITH INDIVIDUAL PATIENTS		SESSIONS WITH FAMILY AND NON-FAMILY GROUPS	
	HOURS PER WEEK	NUMBER PER WEEK	HOURS PER WEEK	NUMBER PER WEEK
ALL PHYSICIANS	35.6	39.2	2.6	3.4
CENSUS DIVISION				
NEW ENGLAND	29.5	30.8	2.8	4.1
MIDDLE ATLANTIC	39.1	41.1	2.1	2.5
EAST NORTH CENTRAL	34.6	44.0	2.8	3.1
WEST NORTH CENTRAL	34.1	38.0	3.3	3.0
SOUTH ATLANTIC	38.8	41.8	3.1	3.7
EAST SOUTH CENTRAL	34.9	43.3	2.4	2.0
WEST SOUTH CENTRAL	38.6	42.9	3.1	4.3
MOUNTAIN	31.2	33.4	2.3	6.2
PACIFIC	32.8	33.6	2.3	3.4
TYPE OF PRACTICE				
SOLO	37.3	40.8	2.6	3.5
NON-SOLO	32.8	36.6	2.7	3.3
LOCATION				
NONMETROPOLITAN	35.6	38.9	2.5	3.2
METROPOLITAN				
LESS THAN 1,000,000	35.7	41.5	3.0	3.9
1,000,000 AND OVER	35.6	35.5	2.3	3.1
EMPLOYMENT STATUS				
SELF-EMPLOYED	38.1	42.8	2.5	3.3
EMPLOYEE	30.7	31.9	2.8	3.5
PHYSICIAN AGE				
LESS THAN 36 YEARS	31.5	35.2	2.9	3.5
36-45 YEARS	36.1	41.1	2.6	3.3
46-55 YEARS	37.6	40.8	3.0	3.6
56-65 YEARS	36.0	38.5	2.5	3.3
66 OR MORE YEARS	30.5	33.0	1.5	3.2

SOURCE: 1ST-4TH QUARTER 1982 AMA SOCIOECONOMIC MONITORING SYSTEM SURVEYS.

*SEE APPENDIX FOR INFORMATION ON DEFINITIONS AND COMPUTATION PROCEDURES.

TABLE 19 (CONTINUED). STANDARD ERROR OF MEAN PATIENT CARE ACTIVITIES PER WEEK: PSYCHIATRY, 1982*

	SESSIONS WITH INDIVIDUAL PATIENTS		SESSIONS WITH FAMILY AND NON-FAMILY GROUPS	
	HOURS PER WEEK	NUMBER PER WEEK	HOURS PER WEEK	NUMBER PER WEEK
ALL PHYSICIANS	0.63	1.07	0.17	0.32
CENSUS DIVISION				
NEW ENGLAND	1.58	2.01	0.58	1.00
MIDDLE ATLANTIC	1.65	2.59	0.30	0.45
EAST NORTH CENTRAL	1.41	3.49	0.45	0.80
WEST NORTH CENTRAL	3.08	4.88	1.12	1.06
SOUTH ATLANTIC	1.50	2.61	0.51	1.01
EAST SOUTH CENTRAL	3.45	6.17	0.70	0.74
WEST SOUTH CENTRAL	1.73	3.26	0.74	1.43
MOUNTAIN	3.41	5.79	0.75	2.07
PACIFIC	1.34	1.94	0.33	0.72
TYPE OF PRACTICE				
SOLO	0.75	1.29	0.22	0.40
NON-SOLO	1.08	1.88	0.30	0.54
LOCATION				
NONMETROPOLITAN	0.80	1.34	0.22	0.41
METROPOLITAN				
LESS THAN 1,000,000	1.27	2.33	0.36	0.60
1,000,000 AND OVER	1.60	2.25	0.41	1.05
EMPLOYMENT STATUS				
SELF-EMPLOYED	0.72	1.31	0.20	0.38
EMPLOYEE	1.09	1.72	0.34	0.61
PHYSICIAN AGE				
LESS THAN 36 YEARS	1.78	3.10	0.41	0.80
36-45 YEARS	1.04	1.76	0.33	0.52
46-55 YEARS	1.25	2.12	0.34	0.67
56-65 YEARS	1.35	2.50	0.35	0.60
66 OR MORE YEARS	2.03	3.26	0.63	1.69

SOURCE: 1ST-4TH QUARTER 1982 AMA SOCIOECONOMIC MONITORING SYSTEM SURVEYS.

*SEE APPENDIX FOR INFORMATION ON DEFINITIONS AND COMPUTATION PROCEDURES.

TABLE 20. MEAN PATIENT CARE ACTIVITIES PER WEEK: RADIOLOGY, 1982*

	READING FILMS		RADIODIAGNOSTIC PROCEDURES		RADIOTHERAPY PATIENTS		CONSULTATIONS	
	HOURS PER WEEK	FILMS READ PER WEEK	HOURS PER WEEK	NUMBER PER WEEK	HOURS PER WEEK	NUMBER PER WEEK	HOURS PER WEEK	NUMBER PER WEEK
ALL PHYSICIANS	26.8	297.5	11.6	42.0	3.4	4.6	5.7	35.2
CENSUS DIVISION								
NEW ENGLAND	24.3	258.1	10.6	28.4	1.9	0.7	5.5	36.0
MIDDLE ATLANTIC	28.5	290.4	11.4	38.9	1.6	3.8	5.1	30.3
EAST NORTH CENTRAL	28.0	293.6	10.3	35.8	4.9	3.9	5.9	40.4
WEST NORTH CENTRAL	30.2	357.5	12.4	45.5	4.7	10.4	5.5	31.4
SOUTH ATLANTIC	25.3	306.9	13.4	54.2	3.2	5.5	7.4	43.8
EAST SOUTH CENTRAL	27.5	369.6	10.8	32.8	4.4	3.1	4.5	31.7
WEST SOUTH CENTRAL	29.6	340.1	13.2	58.9	1.3	1.7	5.5	29.3
MOUNTAIN	23.7	268.3	13.9	34.2	3.7	4.0	4.3	28.6
PACIFIC	24.7	249.5	9.5	34.1	4.8	8.2	5.1	30.9
TYPE OF PRACTICE								
SOLO	23.3	306.4	12.4	38.7	3.0	2.8	5.1	40.8
NON-SOLO	27.2	296.6	11.5	42.3	3.4	4.8	5.8	34.6
LOCATION								
NONMETROPOLITAN	26.6	285.3	11.8	39.9	2.7	4.8	5.9	38.2
METROPOLITAN								
LESS THAN 1,000,000	28.2	328.4	11.8	47.7	3.4	3.3	5.5	30.2
1,000,000 AND OVER	22.9	243.7	9.6	31.5	7.1	8.9	5.4	39.3
EMPLOYMENT STATUS								
SELF-EMPLOYED	28.3	329.4	12.5	48.3	2.5	3.9	5.3	34.4
EMPLOYEE	25.2	261.1	10.6	34.8	4.3	5.5	6.2	36.2
PHYSICIAN AGE								
LESS THAN 36 YEARS	28.5	277.2	12.2	37.6	0.8	3.3	5.7	42.4
36-45 YEARS	27.2	285.7	12.2	43.9	4.2	5.4	6.2	35.2
46-55 YEARS	25.8	303.6	11.5	40.7	4.1	4.5	5.3	35.6
56-65 YEARS	26.0	327.9	10.8	47.9	2.1	4.1	5.8	33.9
66 OR MORE YEARS	29.4	314.8	8.1	23.8	0.7	3.0	4.3	22.9

SOURCE: 1ST-4TH QUARTER 1982 AMA SOCIOECONOMIC MONITORING SYSTEM SURVEYS.

*SEE APPENDIX FOR INFORMATION ON DEFINITIONS AND COMPUTATION PROCEDURES.

TABLE 20 (CONTINUED). STANDARD ERROR OF MEAN PATIENT CARE ACTIVITIES PER WEEK: RADIOLOGY, 1982*

	READING FILMS		RADIODIAGNOSTIC PROCEDURES		RADIOTHERAPY PATIENTS		CONSULTATIONS	
	HOURS PER WEEK	FILMS READ PER WEEK	HOURS PER WEEK	NUMBER PER WEEK	HOURS PER WEEK	NUMBER PER WEEK	HOURS PER WEEK	NUMBER PER WEEK
ALL PHYSICIANS	0.75	13.19	0.46	2.67	0.56	0.97	0.22	2.20
CENSUS DIVISION								
NEW ENGLAND	2.33	30.29	1.18	4.61	1.29	0.66	0.62	8.08
MIDDLE ATLANTIC	1.66	38.37	1.14	5.47	0.68	1.81	0.45	5.34
EAST NORTH CENTRAL	2.04	28.05	1.04	4.26	1.75	1.67	0.56	8.07
WEST NORTH CENTRAL	4.57	74.04	2.52	12.17	2.68	6.22	1.02	5.62
SOUTH ATLANTIC	1.64	29.03	1.11	7.79	1.27	3.26	0.60	5.34
EAST SOUTH CENTRAL	3.45	79.36	1.56	5.14	2.27	1.69	0.44	5.49
WEST SOUTH CENTRAL	2.37	45.40	1.53	14.09	1.14	1.36	0.89	4.35
MOUNTAIN	3.22	57.73	2.73	6.17	2.34	3.14	0.51	3.86
PACIFIC	1.68	27.87	1.00	5.03	1.87	3.46	0.41	4.52
TYPE OF PRACTICE								
SOLO	1.79	49.91	1.54	5.79	1.68	1.50	0.52	6.83
NON-SOLO	0.80	13.53	0.48	2.90	0.60	1.06	0.24	2.33
LOCATION								
NONMETROPOLITAN	0.98	16.97	0.66	3.13	0.68	1.45	0.32	3.53
METROPOLITAN								
LESS THAN 1,000,000	1.30	24.07	0.73	5.48	0.90	1.09	0.36	2.58
1,000,000 AND OVER	2.28	35.83	1.35	5.10	2.67	4.29	0.50	8.36
EMPLOYMENT STATUS								
SELF-EMPLOYED	1.02	20.05	0.63	3.41	0.71	1.22	0.29	2.48
EMPLOYEE	1.09	16.27	0.67	4.30	0.88	1.56	0.34	3.72
PHYSICIAN AGE								
LESS THAN 36 YEARS	2.07	29.10	1.35	4.53	0.73	3.63	0.79	9.56
36-45 YEARS	1.34	19.66	0.73	4.01	0.99	1.82	0.38	2.64
46-55 YEARS	1.25	26.11	0.91	5.14	1.16	1.41	0.37	5.22
56-65 YEARS	1.68	33.83	1.09	9.74	1.05	1.88	0.49	4.04
66 OR MORE YEARS	2.78	84.24	1.12	4.51	0.41	1.97	0.71	4.95

SOURCE: 1ST-4TH QUARTER 1982 AMA SOCIOECONOMIC MONITORING SYSTEM SURVEYS.

*SEE APPENDIX FOR INFORMATION ON DEFINITIONS AND COMPUTATION PROCEDURES.

TABLE 21. MEAN PATIENT CARE ACTIVITIES PER WEEK: ANESTHESIOLOGY, 1982*

	PATIENTS ANESTHETIZED PERSONALLY BY PHYSICIAN		PATIENTS ANESTHETIZED BY NURSE ANESTHETISTS SUPERVISED BY PHYSICIAN		PRE-ANESTHESIA AND OTHER INPATIENT VISITS	
	HOURS PER WEEK	NUMBER PER WEEK	HOURS SUPERVISING PER WEEK	NUMBER PER WEEK	HOURS PER WEEK	NUMBER PER WEEK
ALL PHYSICIANS	31.3	18.2	8.8	36.1	11.0	13.7
CENSUS DIVISION						
NEW ENGLAND	27.5	16.1	8.7	34.3	16.5	17.2
MIDDLE ATLANTIC	28.1	15.7	10.1	41.1	13.6	16.0
EAST NORTH CENTRAL	28.0	17.0	8.3	34.3	10.5	13.4
WEST NORTH CENTRAL	20.4	15.7	6.1	31.9	23.1	24.1
SOUTH ATLANTIC	31.6	19.3	9.3	37.2	12.3	18.5
EAST SOUTH CENTRAL	32.1	18.3	9.0	40.0	14.6	12.3
WEST SOUTH CENTRAL	32.5	19.5	9.3	45.5	12.2	21.2
MOUNTAIN	41.1	22.0	7.2	33.1	3.8	5.2
PACIFIC	38.8	20.6	9.2	31.5	2.5	1.9
TYPE OF PRACTICE						
SOLO	36.0	20.8	9.4	38.1	3.4	5.7
NON-SOLO	28.9	16.9	8.6	35.1	14.7	17.6
LOCATION						
NONMETROPOLITAN	29.5	17.5	9.0	36.4	11.9	14.2
METROPOLITAN						
LESS THAN 1,000,000	33.2	18.9	8.7	37.3	11.1	15.1
1,000,000 AND OVER	31.4	18.3	8.7	30.5	7.5	7.0
EMPLOYMENT STATUS						
SELF-EMPLOYED	33.5	19.9	9.1	37.4	8.7	11.2
EMPLOYEE	27.2	14.9	8.4	33.7	15.1	18.4
PHYSICIAN AGE						
LESS THAN 36 YEARS	28.9	15.6	7.6	34.5	16.9	23.3
36-45 YEARS	30.6	18.4	8.6	36.6	11.8	13.5
46-55 YEARS	32.0	18.9	9.0	33.3	8.0	12.2
56-65 YEARS	32.5	18.3	9.5	39.1	10.8	11.3
66 OR MORE YEARS	33.9	18.7	9.4	37.2	5.5	9.4

SOURCE: 1ST-4TH QUARTER 1982 AMA SOCIOECONOMIC MONITORING SYSTEM SURVEYS.

*SEE APPENDIX FOR INFORMATION ON DEFINITIONS AND COMPUTATION PROCEDURES.

TABLE 21 (CONTINUED). STANDARD ERROR OF MEAN PATIENT CARE ACTIVITIES PER WEEK: ANESTHESIOLOGY, 1982*

	PATIENTS ANESTHETIZED PERSONALLY BY PHYSICIAN		PATIENTS ANESTHETIZED BY NURSE ANESTHETISTS SUPERVISED BY PHYSICIAN		PRE-ANESTHESIA AND OTHER INPATIENT VISITS	
	HOURS PER WEEK	NUMBER PER WEEK	HOURS SUPERVISING PER WEEK	NUMBER PER WEEK	HOURS PER WEEK	NUMBER PER WEEK
ALL PHYSICIANS	0.96	0.57	0.30	1.33	0.82	1.36
CENSUS DIVISION						
NEW ENGLAND	3.05	1.52	0.78	2.95	2.38	3.35
MIDDLE ATLANTIC	2.51	1.62	0.95	5.05	2.30	3.61
EAST NORTH CENTRAL	1.82	1.19	0.67	2.89	1.86	3.35
WEST NORTH CENTRAL	4.16	3.54	0.92	3.66	3.66	3.95
SOUTH ATLANTIC	2.47	1.61	0.88	3.41	1.91	4.19
EAST SOUTH CENTRAL	6.53	3.15	1.38	4.72	6.16	5.04
WEST SOUTH CENTRAL	3.68	2.08	0.96	4.60	2.98	6.11
MOUNTAIN	2.97	1.86	0.74	3.68	1.97	2.94
PACIFIC	1.79	0.93	0.76	2.21	0.97	1.11
TYPE OF PRACTICE						
SOLO	1.48	0.79	0.55	2.32	0.89	1.87
NON-SOLO	1.20	0.74	0.36	1.62	1.06	1.75
LOCATION						
NONMETROPOLITAN	1.54	0.91	0.46	2.09	1.29	1.98
METROPOLITAN						
LESS THAN 1,000,000	1.37	0.86	0.47	1.97	1.18	2.26
1,000,000 AND OVER	2.40	1.27	0.81	3.06	2.35	2.83
EMPLOYMENT STATUS						
SELF-EMPLOYED	1.13	0.68	0.37	1.51	0.98	1.60
EMPLOYEE	1.66	0.97	0.52	2.52	1.42	2.43
PHYSICIAN AGE						
LESS THAN 36 YEARS	3.53	2.13	0.88	3.85	2.97	6.00
36-45 YEARS	1.68	0.96	0.44	2.19	1.47	2.15
46-55 YEARS	1.78	1.04	0.62	2.00	1.26	2.57
56-65 YEARS	1.72	1.10	0.74	3.32	1.61	2.11
66 OR MORE YEARS	2.97	1.31	1.60	8.14	2.65	5.18

SOURCE: 1ST-4TH QUARTER 1982 AMA SOCIOECONOMIC MONITORING SYSTEM SURVEYS.

*SEE APPENDIX FOR INFORMATION ON DEFINITIONS AND COMPUTATION PROCEDURES.

TABLE 22. MEAN PATIENT CARE ACTIVITIES PER WEEK: PATHOLOGY, 1982*

	SURGICAL CONSULTATIONS		EXAMINATIONS OF SURGICAL SPECIMENS		LABORATORY PROCEDURES		AUTOPSIES	
	HOURS PER WEEK	NUMBER PER WEEK	HOURS PER WEEK	NUMBER PER WEEK	HOURS PER WEEK	NUMBER PER WEEK	HOURS PER WEEK	NUMBER PER WEEK
ALL PHYSICIANS	4.2	1.3	15.4	79.4	6.5	33.7	4.2	1.3
CENSUS DIVISION								
NEW ENGLAND	3.8	1.4	16.1	95.7	3.5	15.3	3.8	1.4
MIDDLE ATLANTIC	6.4	2.2	16.3	55.9	7.2	22.5	6.4	2.2
EAST NORTH CENTRAL	4.1	0.9	13.6	89.1	9.0	47.8	4.1	0.9
WEST NORTH CENTRAL	3.7	1.2	16.3	60.3	6.9	35.2	3.7	1.2
SOUTH ATLANTIC	3.3	0.9	15.5	68.7	6.3	51.9	3.3	0.9
EAST SOUTH CENTRAL	3.8	1.3	17.8	128.6	6.8	44.7	3.8	1.3
WEST SOUTH CENTRAL	1.1	0.5	14.3	86.2	5.1	36.2	1.1	0.5
MOUNTAIN	6.2	1.7	12.5	104.2	6.8	29.6	6.2	1.7
PACIFIC	4.3	1.3	15.8	83.6	4.5	11.5	4.3	1.3
TYPE OF PRACTICE								
SOLO	3.7	1.2	15.7	78.7	6.6	25.5	3.7	1.2
NON-SOLO	4.3	1.3	15.3	79.5	6.5	35.2	4.3	1.3
LOCATION								
NONMETROPOLITAN	4.5	1.2	15.3	69.0	6.6	24.3	4.5	1.2
METROPOLITAN								
LESS THAN 1,000,000	4.0	1.4	15.5	86.7	6.2	28.5	4.0	1.4
1,000,000 AND OVER	4.0	1.0	15.2	92.4	8.4	111.7	4.0	1.0
EMPLOYMENT STATUS								
SELF-EMPLOYED	3.8	1.6	15.7	84.7	6.7	36.8	3.8	1.6
EMPLOYEE	4.4	1.1	15.2	76.5	6.4	32.1	4.4	1.1
PHYSICIAN AGE								
LESS THAN 36 YEARS	4.1	1.1	19.0	78.1	4.8	23.6	4.1	1.1
36-45 YEARS	3.7	0.9	15.4	74.5	7.5	37.3	3.7	0.9
46-55 YEARS	4.0	1.7	15.1	87.0	7.5	46.7	4.0	1.7
56-65 YEARS	6.2	1.6	13.8	82.1	3.9	14.8	6.2	1.6
66 OR MORE YEARS	2.7	0.8	15.5	51.0	5.6	4.5	2.7	0.8

SOURCE: 1ST-4TH QUARTER 1982 AMA SOCIOECONOMIC MONITORING SYSTEM SURVEYS.

*SEE APPENDIX FOR INFORMATION ON DEFINITIONS AND COMPUTATION PROCEDURES.

TABLE 22 (CONTINUED). STANDARD ERROR OF MEAN PATIENT CARE ACTIVITIES PER WEEK: PATHOLOGY, 1982*

	SURGICAL CONSULTATIONS		EXAMINATIONS OF SURGICAL SPECIMENS		LABORATORY PROCEDURES		AUTOPSIES	
	HOURS PER WEEK	NUMBER PER WEEK	HOURS PER WEEK	NUMBER PER WEEK	HOURS PER WEEK	NUMBER PER WEEK	HOURS PER WEEK	NUMBER PER WEEK
ALL PHYSICIANS	0.35	0.15	0.67	4.14	0.46	5.81	0.35	0.15
CENSUS DIVISION								
NEW ENGLAND	0.81	0.31	1.58	19.18	1.10	7.89	0.81	0.31
MIDDLE ATLANTIC	1.10	0.63	2.22	7.49	1.11	6.29	1.10	0.63
EAST NORTH CENTRAL	0.92	0.17	1.34	9.35	1.60	18.19	0.92	0.17
WEST NORTH CENTRAL	0.74	0.24	1.74	10.08	1.19	11.11	0.74	0.24
SOUTH ATLANTIC	0.60	0.19	1.58	8.66	1.05	24.47	0.60	0.19
EAST SOUTH CENTRAL	1.32	0.47	2.22	17.25	1.56	19.61	1.32	0.47
WEST SOUTH CENTRAL	0.46	0.17	2.10	20.84	1.14	21.20	0.46	0.17
MOUNTAIN	2.49	0.38	2.64	23.49	2.62	18.25	2.49	0.38
PACIFIC	0.89	0.33	2.03	10.49	1.01	3.75	0.89	0.33
TYPE OF PRACTICE								
SOLO	0.81	0.25	1.59	10.83	1.15	7.80	0.81	0.25
NON-SOLO	0.39	0.17	0.74	4.49	0.51	6.73	0.39	0.17
LOCATION								
NONMETROPOLITAN	0.61	0.16	0.87	5.60	0.72	4.61	0.61	0.16
METROPOLITAN								
LESS THAN 1,000,000	0.44	0.26	1.09	6.42	0.62	5.92	0.44	0.26
1,000,000 AND OVER	1.24	0.30	1.99	13.70	2.09	53.26	1.24	0.30
EMPLOYMENT STATUS								
SELF-EMPLOYED	0.42	0.37	1.04	6.64	0.81	8.75	0.42	0.37
EMPLOYEE	0.48	0.12	0.86	5.27	0.57	7.57	0.48	0.12
PHYSICIAN AGE								
LESS THAN 36 YEARS	1.00	0.30	3.72	12.05	0.87	10.84	1.00	0.30
36-45 YEARS	0.50	0.12	0.99	7.23	0.91	12.82	0.50	0.12
46-55 YEARS	0.60	0.38	1.00	7.18	0.79	10.38	0.60	0.38
56-65 YEARS	1.15	0.24	1.54	9.97	0.91	5.24	1.15	0.24
66 OR MORE YEARS	0.94	0.32	3.20	14.73	1.87	2.23	0.94	0.32

SOURCE: 1ST-4TH QUARTER 1982 AMA SOCIOECONOMIC MONITORING SYSTEM SURVEYS.

*SEE APPENDIX FOR INFORMATION ON DEFINITIONS AND COMPUTATION PROCEDURES.

TABLE 23. MEAN NUMBER OF DAYS WAITING TIME TO BE SCHEDULED FOR AN APPOINTMENT, 1982*

	ALL PHYSICIANS**	SPECIALTY				
		GENERAL & FAMILY PRACTICE	INTERNAL MEDICINE	SURGERY	PEDIATRICS	OBSTETRICS/ GYNECOLOGY
ALL PHYSICIANS	6.9	3.5	7.9	8.4	5.0	12.3
CENSUS DIVISION						
NEW ENGLAND	7.9	4.2	9.3	7.0	10.3	11.0
MIDDLE ATLANTIC	7.0	3.3	8.0	9.5	5.5	7.6
EAST NORTH CENTRAL	6.8	3.2	6.6	9.6	3.9	13.5
WEST NORTH CENTRAL	9.5	3.9	9.4	18.9	4.4	14.2
SOUTH ATLANTIC	6.8	5.1	6.8	7.5	5.4	11.7
EAST SOUTH CENTRAL	4.9	1.5	7.7	4.7	5.5	5.6
WEST SOUTH CENTRAL	5.0	2.2	7.0	5.2	2.5	12.6
MOUNTAIN	6.0	2.9	10.3	6.4	5.2	12.3
PACIFIC	7.7	4.4	8.9	7.9	4.1	18.9
TYPE OF PRACTICE						
SOLO	6.2	3.2	6.6	8.2	4.7	7.8
NON-SOLO	7.6	4.0	9.0	8.7	5.2	17.0
LOCATION						
NONMETROPOLITAN	6.6	3.8	7.8	7.6	4.8	14.0
METROPOLITAN						
LESS THAN 1,000,000	7.9	3.2	9.1	10.1	5.8	11.9
1,000,000 AND OVER	5.4	2.6	4.9	6.9	3.8	6.5
EMPLOYMENT STATUS						
SELF-EMPLOYED	6.8	3.5	7.1	8.9	5.0	9.9
EMPLOYEE	7.1	3.6	9.2	7.2	5.0	18.8
PHYSICIAN AGE						
LESS THAN 36 YEARS	4.5	3.4	5.3	5.7	3.3	7.8
36-45 YEARS	7.5	5.3	8.3	8.0	5.2	13.0
46-55 YEARS	8.7	4.3	8.2	10.7	4.5	17.2
56-65 YEARS	6.2	2.5	9.1	6.9	7.0	10.0
66 OR MORE YEARS	5.6	2.5	9.7	8.4	5.1	6.5

SOURCE: 1982 AMA SOCIOECONOMIC MONITORING SYSTEM CORE SURVEY.

*SEE APPENDIX FOR INFORMATION ON DEFINITIONS AND COMPUTATION PROCEDURES.
**EXCLUDES RADIOLOGY, ANESTHESIOLOGY AND PATHOLOGY, BUT OTHERWISE INCLUDES SPECIALTIES NOT LISTED SEPARATELY.

TABLE 23 (CONTINUED). STANDARD ERROR OF THE MEAN NUMBER OF DAYS WAITING TIME TO BE SCHEDULED FOR AN APPOINTMENT, 1982*

	ALL PHYSICIANS**	SPECIALTY				
		GENERAL & FAMILY PRACTICE	INTERNAL MEDICINE	SURGERY	PEDIATRICS	OBSTETRICS/ GYNECOLOGY
ALL PHYSICIANS	0.28	0.27	0.48	0.75	0.53	1.62
CENSUS DIVISION						
NEW ENGLAND	0.74	1.01	1.97	1.50	3.76	2.35
MIDDLE ATLANTIC	0.55	0.69	1.37	1.36	1.27	1.32
EAST NORTH CENTRAL	0.48	0.46	0.82	1.21	0.79	2.80
WEST NORTH CENTRAL	2.46	0.78	1.88	9.57	1.66	7.23
SOUTH ATLANTIC	0.55	0.86	0.78	1.55	1.54	1.98
EAST SOUTH CENTRAL	0.58	0.35	1.52	1.09	2.12	1.16
WEST SOUTH CENTRAL	0.47	0.38	1.23	0.86	0.86	2.99
MOUNTAIN	0.86	0.84	3.52	1.33	2.56	4.26
PACIFIC	0.90	1.10	1.48	1.06	0.94	8.93
TYPE OF PRACTICE						
SOLO	0.41	0.33	0.72	1.28	0.78	0.71
NON-SOLO	0.39	0.44	0.65	0.74	0.71	3.17
LOCATION						
NONMETROPOLITAN	0.34	0.35	0.71	0.62	0.69	3.04
METROPOLITAN						
LESS THAN 1,000,000	0.60	0.45	0.86	1.85	1.01	1.64
1,000,000 AND OVER	0.45	0.58	0.79	0.92	1.23	1.05
EMPLOYMENT STATUS						
SELF-EMPLOYED	0.35	0.30	0.61	1.00	0.64	1.08
EMPLOYEE	0.48	0.59	0.79	0.61	0.91	5.25
PHYSICIAN AGE						
LESS THAN 36 YEARS	0.35	0.61	0.74	0.98	1.12	1.46
36-45 YEARS	0.39	0.93	0.81	0.67	0.83	1.91
46-55 YEARS	0.93	0.64	0.95	2.27	0.89	5.39
56-65 YEARS	0.41	0.24	1.30	0.94	1.82	1.74
66 OR MORE YEARS	0.70	0.41	2.86	2.14	2.05	1.26

SOURCE: 1982 AMA SOCIOECONOMIC MONITORING SYSTEM CORE SURVEY.

*SEE APPENDIX FOR INFORMATION ON DEFINITIONS AND COMPUTATION PROCEDURES.
**EXCLUDES RADIOLOGY, ANESTHESIOLOGY AND PATHOLOGY, BUT OTHERWISE INCLUDES SPECIALTIES NOT LISTED SEPARATELY.

TABLE 24. MEAN NUMBER OF MINUTES WAITING TIME BY PATIENTS ARRIVING FOR AN APPOINTMENT, 1982*

	ALL PHYSICIANS**	SPECIALTY				
		GENERAL & FAMILY PRACTICE	INTERNAL MEDICINE	SURGERY	PEDIATRICS	OBSTETRICS/ GYNECOLOGY
ALL PHYSICIANS	19.2	22.9	18.6	21.0	19.7	22.0
CENSUS DIVISION						
NEW ENGLAND	15.4	15.5	15.4	21.7	18.5	18.9
MIDDLE ATLANTIC	19.0	23.8	19.5	22.8	17.5	18.1
EAST NORTH CENTRAL	19.7	25.8	19.1	21.2	20.5	22.7
WEST NORTH CENTRAL	21.2	20.0	22.9	24.0	24.2	20.9
SOUTH ATLANTIC	19.4	21.3	18.3	22.0	18.3	25.3
EAST SOUTH CENTRAL	21.7	24.0	20.3	18.8	18.8	32.8
WEST SOUTH CENTRAL	22.5	27.1	20.1	21.8	26.0	21.7
MOUNTAIN	17.9	19.4	12.8	18.9	25.4	21.7
PACIFIC	16.9	22.4	17.1	17.6	18.6	17.8
TYPE OF PRACTICE						
SOLO	18.4	23.2	17.7	19.7	19.7	21.6
NON-SOLO	20.1	22.5	19.3	22.3	19.7	22.5
LOCATION						
NONMETROPOLITAN	19.4	23.4	18.6	21.0	18.9	23.4
METROPOLITAN						
LESS THAN 1,000,000	19.4	20.0	18.1	22.1	20.5	21.5
1,000,000 AND OVER	18.0	30.3	19.5	17.9	20.8	18.3
EMPLOYMENT STATUS						
SELF-EMPLOYED	18.9	23.6	18.0	20.4	19.3	19.7
EMPLOYEE	19.9	20.7	19.6	22.5	20.3	28.6
PHYSICIAN AGE						
LESS THAN 36 YEARS	19.1	21.6	18.5	20.5	17.3	19.6
36-45 YEARS	19.6	23.1	19.9	21.3	21.0	21.8
46-55 YEARS	18.8	21.6	17.5	21.2	22.9	23.3
56-65 YEARS	18.3	21.4	18.1	20.3	16.6	21.7
66 OR MORE YEARS	21.2	27.1	16.7	20.6	16.3	23.0

SOURCE: 1982 AMA SOCIOECONOMIC MONITORING SYSTEM CORE SURVEY.

*SEE APPENDIX FOR INFORMATION ON DEFINITIONS AND COMPUTATION PROCEDURES.
**EXCLUDES RADIOLOGY, ANESTHESIOLOGY AND PATHOLOGY, BUT OTHERWISE INCLUDES SPECIALTIES NOT LISTED SEPARATELY.

TABLE 24 (CONTINUED). STANDARD ERROR OF THE MEAN NUMBER OF MINUTES WAITING TIME BY PATIENTS ARRIVING FOR AN APPOINTMENT, 1982*

SPECIALTY

	ALL PHYSICIANS**	GENERAL & FAMILY PRACTICE	INTERNAL MEDICINE	SURGERY	PEDIATRICS	OBSTETRICS/ GYNECOLOGY
ALL PHYSICIANS	0.32	0.80	0.62	0.56	0.93	1.09
CENSUS DIVISION						
NEW ENGLAND	1.07	1.70	1.98	2.81	4.41	2.04
MIDDLE ATLANTIC	0.79	2.57	1.38	1.39	1.94	2.06
EAST NORTH CENTRAL	0.89	2.83	1.56	1.48	2.75	2.67
WEST NORTH CENTRAL	1.07	1.75	2.56	2.33	5.11	3.77
SOUTH ATLANTIC	0.75	1.54	1.42	1.58	2.00	2.36
EAST SOUTH CENTRAL	1.47	3.01	2.10	1.70	2.52	9.23
WEST SOUTH CENTRAL	1.31	1.99	3.56	1.72	3.62	2.85
MOUNTAIN	1.06	2.02	2.24	1.67	5.31	4.14
PACIFIC	0.63	1.92	1.18	1.11	1.84	1.73
TYPE OF PRACTICE						
SOLO	0.48	1.16	0.85	0.86	1.57	1.82
NON-SOLO	0.42	1.05	0.90	0.71	1.16	1.13
LOCATION						
NONMETROPOLITAN	0.46	1.05	0.93	0.82	1.32	1.94
METROPOLITAN						
LESS THAN 1,000,000	0.51	1.07	0.91	0.95	1.57	1.24
1,000,000 AND OVER	0.84	4.27	1.81	1.10	2.43	2.07
EMPLOYMENT STATUS						
SELF-EMPLOYED	0.37	0.97	0.73	0.67	1.16	0.92
EMPLOYEE	0.63	1.29	1.16	1.00	1.54	3.13
PHYSICIAN AGE						
LESS THAN 36 YEARS	0.95	1.79	1.45	2.05	2.30	2.47
36-45 YEARS	0.52	1.32	1.17	0.81	1.51	1.41
46-55 YEARS	0.63	1.55	1.17	1.06	2.38	2.84
56-65 YEARS	0.62	1.21	1.36	1.31	1.61	1.83
66 OR MORE YEARS	1.40	2.94	2.24	2.59	2.60	4.59

SOURCE: 1982 AMA SOCIOECONOMIC MONITORING SYSTEM CORE SURVEY.

*SEE APPENDIX FOR INFORMATION ON DEFINITIONS AND COMPUTATION PROCEDURES.
**EXCLUDES RADIOLOGY, ANESTHESIOLOGY AND PATHOLOGY, BUT OTHERWISE INCLUDES SPECIALTIES NOT LISTED SEPARATELY.

TABLE 25.   MEAN NUMBER OF PATIENTS DISCHARGED FROM THE HOSPITAL PER WEEK, 1982*

SPECIALTY

	ALL PHYSICIANS**	GENERAL & FAMILY PRACTICE	INTERNAL MEDICINE	SURGERY	PEDIATRICS	OBSTETRICS/ GYNECOLOGY
ALL PHYSICIANS	5.8	5.7	5.4	7.5	7.1	8.9
CENSUS DIVISION						
NEW ENGLAND	3.8	4.4	5.0	5.0	3.6	.
MIDDLE ATLANTIC	5.0	3.4	4.3	5.7	5.2	8.1
EAST NORTH CENTRAL	6.9	8.0	6.3	8.7	8.8	10.7
WEST NORTH CENTRAL	6.8	7.9	6.4	9.4	5.4	.
SOUTH ATLANTIC	5.8	4.1	6.4	7.7	5.8	9.5
EAST SOUTH CENTRAL	7.4	6.9	5.8	8.4	12.8	9.5
WEST SOUTH CENTRAL	7.9	7.7	6.7	10.9	9.5	10.8
MOUNTAIN	5.0	4.0	4.7	7.6	13.9	.
PACIFIC	4.0	3.7	3.5	5.2	5.0	7.8
TYPE OF PRACTICE						
SOLO	5.2	5.1	5.4	6.8	6.9	7.1
NON-SOLO	6.4	6.6	5.4	8.1	7.2	10.1
LOCATION						
NONMETROPOLITAN	5.7	5.8	5.4	7.3	6.9	9.5
METROPOLITAN						
LESS THAN 1,000,000	6.5	6.2	5.9	8.0	8.9	9.1
1,000,000 AND OVER	4.1	3.7	4.2	6.3	3.6	6.0
EMPLOYMENT STATUS						
SELF-EMPLOYED	6.1	6.0	5.8	7.5	8.4	9.1
EMPLOYEE	4.9	4.4	4.3	7.6	4.2	8.5
PHYSICIAN AGE						
LESS THAN 36 YEARS	5.6	6.2	5.1	6.2	7.4	10.6
36-45 YEARS	5.9	6.1	6.1	7.8	5.8	9.0
46-55 YEARS	6.3	6.3	5.8	8.0	5.9	8.7
56-65 YEARS	6.2	5.9	4.4	8.3	10.4	8.9
66 OR MORE YEARS	4.0	3.7	3.7	3.9		7.0

SOURCE: 3RD AND 4TH QUARTER 1982 AMA SOCIOECONOMIC MONITORING SYSTEM SURVEYS.

 *SEE APPENDIX FOR INFORMATION ON DEFINITIONS AND COMPUTATION PROCEDURES.
**EXCLUDES RADIOLOGY, ANESTHESIOLOGY AND PATHOLOGY, BUT OTHERWISE INCLUDES SPECIALTIES NOT LISTED SEPARATELY.
  . INDICATES FEWER THAN TEN OBSERVATIONS.

TABLE 25 (CONTINUED). STANDARD ERROR OF THE MEAN NUMBER OF PATIENTS DISCHARGED FROM THE HOSPITAL PER WEEK, 1982*

	ALL PHYSICIANS**	SPECIALTY GENERAL & FAMILY PRACTICE	INTERNAL MEDICINE	SURGERY	PEDIATRICS	OBSTETRICS/ GYNECOLOGY
ALL PHYSICIANS	0.17	0.31	0.30	0.35	0.68	0.53
CENSUS DIVISION						
NEW ENGLAND	0.42	1.05	1.17	0.76	1.21	
MIDDLE ATLANTIC	0.46	0.84	0.53	0.57	1.14	1.03
EAST NORTH CENTRAL	0.49	0.85	0.84	1.16	2.18	1.47
WEST NORTH CENTRAL	0.66	0.92	1.66	1.93	0.95	
SOUTH ATLANTIC	0.37	0.79	0.85	0.71	1.08	1.47
EAST SOUTH CENTRAL	0.64	0.86	1.74	1.15	2.71	1.58
WEST SOUTH CENTRAL	0.56	1.12	0.92	1.32	1.98	1.31
MOUNTAIN	0.73	0.75	1.10	0.89	5.28	.
PACIFIC	0.28	0.56	0.43	0.51	1.05	1.55
TYPE OF PRACTICE						
SOLO	0.21	0.42	0.46	0.48	0.83	0.75
NON-SOLO	0.25	0.46	0.39	0.49	0.99	0.73
LOCATION						
NONMETROPOLITAN	0.23	0.42	0.40	0.51	1.12	0.81
METROPOLITAN						
LESS THAN 1,000,000	0.30	0.56	0.54	0.55	0.94	0.80
1,000,000 AND OVER	0.37	0.74	0.74	0.90	0.97	1.32
EMPLOYMENT STATUS						
SELF-EMPLOYED	0.18	0.36	0.35	0.35	0.86	0.59
EMPLOYEE	0.39	0.60	0.55	0.97	0.81	1.25
PHYSICIAN AGE						
LESS THAN 36 YEARS	0.42	0.69	0.64	1.22	1.80	1.61
36-45 YEARS	0.27	0.60	0.52	0.55	0.77	0.95
46-55 YEARS	0.41	0.81	0.75	0.74	0.82	1.24
56-65 YEARS	0.39	0.61	0.64	0.76	2.32	1.23
66 OR MORE YEARS	0.39	0.73	0.74	0.76	.	1.60

SOURCE: 3RD AND 4TH QUARTER 1982 AMA SOCIOECONOMIC MONITORING SYSTEM SURVEYS.

*SEE APPENDIX FOR INFORMATION ON DEFINITIONS AND COMPUTATION PROCEDURES.
**EXCLUDES RADIOLOGY, ANESTHESIOLOGY AND PATHOLOGY, BUT OTHERWISE INCLUDES SPECIALTIES NOT LISTED SEPARATELY.
. INDICATES FEWER THAN TEN OBSERVATIONS.

TABLE 26. MEAN NUMBER OF DAYS FOR HOSPITAL STAYS PER PATIENT, 1982*

	ALL PHYSICIANS**	SPECIALTY				
		GENERAL & FAMILY PRACTICE	INTERNAL MEDICINE	SURGERY	PEDIATRICS	OBSTETRICS/ GYNECOLOGY
ALL PHYSICIANS	6.6	5.9	7.3	4.9	4.1	3.8
CENSUS DIVISION						
NEW ENGLAND	7.0		7.3	4.5	4.0	
MIDDLE ATLANTIC	7.8	9.0	9.6	5.5	4.0	3.7
EAST NORTH CENTRAL	7.8	6.4	7.7	5.5	4.6	3.7
WEST NORTH CENTRAL	7.3	5.4	6.0	6.5	6.0	.
SOUTH ATLANTIC	6.5	5.4	6.2	4.6	3.7	4.3
EAST SOUTH CENTRAL	6.1	5.3	6.5	4.6	6.0	4.1
WEST SOUTH CENTRAL	6.5	8.1	5.9	4.8	3.9	3.7
MOUNTAIN	4.9	4.4	5.3	5.8	3.1	.
PACIFIC	5.0	4.3	6.8	3.6	3.0	3.4
TYPE OF PRACTICE						
SOLO	6.8	6.1	7.5	4.4	4.2	3.9
NON-SOLO	6.6	5.6	7.1	5.3	4.1	3.7
LOCATION						
NONMETROPOLITAN	6.7	5.9	7.0	4.8	4.4	3.8
METROPOLITAN						
LESS THAN 1,000,000	6.4	5.8	7.0	5.0	3.8	3.8
1,000,000 AND OVER	7.3	6.4	8.6	4.7	4.2	3.8
EMPLOYMENT STATUS						
SELF-EMPLOYED	6.1	5.8	7.3	4.8	3.8	3.8
EMPLOYEE	8.8	6.6	7.1	5.3	5.2	3.7
PHYSICIAN AGE						
LESS THAN 36 YEARS	7.2	4.9	7.1	4.7	3.7	3.5
36-45 YEARS	6.5	6.0	6.7	4.6	4.3	3.6
46-55 YEARS	6.9	5.8	8.0	5.0	3.4	3.6
56-65 YEARS	6.3	5.3	7.4	5.2	4.6	4.3
66 OR MORE YEARS	6.8	8.3	8.5	5.1	.	3.9

*SEE APPENDIX FOR INFORMATION ON DEFINITIONS AND COMPUTATION PROCEDURES.
**EXCLUDES RADIOLOGY, ANESTHESIOLOGY AND PATHOLOGY, BUT OTHERWISE INCLUDES SPECIALTIES NOT LISTED SEPARATELY.
. INDICATES FEWER THAN TEN OBSERVATIONS.

TABLE 26 (CONTINUED). STANDARD ERROR OF THE MEAN NUMBER OF DAYS FOR HOSPITAL STAYS PER PATIENT, 1982*

	ALL PHYSICIANS**	SPECIALTY				
		GENERAL & FAMILY PRACTICE	INTERNAL MEDICINE	SURGERY	PEDIATRICS	OBSTETRICS/ GYNECOLOGY
ALL PHYSICIANS	0.24	0.35	0.21	0.16	0.30	0.10
CENSUS DIVISION						
NEW ENGLAND	0.78	.	0.75	0.53	0.56	.
MIDDLE ATLANTIC	0.65	1.66	0.67	0.42	0.51	0.25
EAST NORTH CENTRAL	0.62	0.44	0.34	0.39	0.55	0.29
WEST NORTH CENTRAL	1.02	0.42	0.54	1.40	2.69	.
SOUTH ATLANTIC	0.63	0.33	0.38	0.32	0.25	0.24
EAST SOUTH CENTRAL	0.81	0.27	0.41	0.48	2.19	0.35
WEST SOUTH CENTRAL	0.74	2.48	0.30	0.38	0.27	0.15
MOUNTAIN	0.30	0.34	0.89	0.53	0.18	.
PACIFIC	0.46	0.24	0.56	0.22	0.26	0.30
TYPE OF PRACTICE						
SOLO	0.36	0.35	0.38	0.18	0.53	0.17
NON-SOLO	0.32	0.65	0.22	0.26	0.37	0.13
LOCATION						
NONMETROPOLITAN	0.34	0.54	0.28	0.26	0.61	0.14
METROPOLITAN						
LESS THAN 1,000,000	0.36	0.43	0.32	0.22	0.22	0.16
1,000,000 AND OVER	0.77	0.96	0.69	0.43	0.59	0.32
EMPLOYMENT STATUS						
SELF-EMPLOYED	0.20	0.24	0.25	0.18	0.28	0.11
EMPLOYEE	0.85	2.07	0.37	0.37	0.96	0.26
PHYSICIAN AGE						
LESS THAN 36 YEARS	0.77	0.28	0.59	0.48	0.29	0.22
36-45 YEARS	0.41	1.24	0.24	0.21	0.61	0.17
46-55 YEARS	0.57	0.74	0.57	0.43	0.26	0.30
56-65 YEARS	0.42	0.20	0.58	0.31	0.89	0.18
66 OR MORE YEARS	0.40	0.82	0.74	0.48	.	0.34

*SEE APPENDIX FOR INFORMATION ON DEFINITIONS AND COMPUTATION PROCEDURES.
**EXCLUDES RADIOLOGY, ANESTHESIOLOGY AND PATHOLOGY, BUT OTHERWISE INCLUDES SPECIALTIES NOT LISTED SEPARATELY.
. INDICATES FEWER THAN TEN OBSERVATIONS.

TABLE 27. MEAN FEE FOR AN OFFICE VISIT WITH AN ESTABLISHED PATIENT (IN DOLLARS), 1982*

	ALL PHYSICIANS**	SPECIALTY				
		GENERAL & FAMILY PRACTICE	INTERNAL MEDICINE	SURGERY	PEDIATRICS	OBSTETRICS/ GYNECOLOGY
ALL PHYSICIANS	21.60	17.48	25.30	23.57	21.10	25.76
CENSUS DIVISION						
NEW ENGLAND	22.37	17.89	24.56	24.46	20.22	24.71
MIDDLE ATLANTIC	24.17	17.45	27.58	26.19	21.90	32.83
EAST NORTH CENTRAL	19.44	16.19	21.56	21.82	19.26	23.52
WEST NORTH CENTRAL	16.99	14.74	19.60	19.73	18.12	19.81
SOUTH ATLANTIC	21.75	16.77	27.03	22.09	20.05	28.26
EAST SOUTH CENTRAL	19.03	16.40	23.69	20.96	18.56	23.26
WEST SOUTH CENTRAL	20.78	17.21	24.25	23.11	21.35	23.14
MOUNTAIN	21.20	18.81	23.18	24.15	19.97	19.86
PACIFIC	25.77	23.19	28.96	27.36	25.65	25.82
TYPE OF PRACTICE						
SOLO	21.15	17.50	24.49	23.52	20.89	25.92
NON-SOLO	22.10	17.45	26.18	23.62	21.26	25.66
LOCATION						
NONMETROPOLITAN	20.76	16.99	23.62	23.41	21.30	25.23
METROPOLITAN						
LESS THAN 1,000,000	21.19	17.57	25.14	22.30	20.07	24.80
1,000,000 AND OVER	27.89	22.71	30.77	30.02	23.59	31.88
EMPLOYMENT STATUS						
SELF-EMPLOYED	21.54	17.50	25.20	23.59	21.13	25.91
EMPLOYEE	21.89	17.32	25.72	23.49	20.98	25.06
PHYSICIAN AGE						
LESS THAN 36 YEARS	21.27	17.51	24.43	25.33	20.05	24.87
36-45 YEARS	22.24	18.47	25.32	22.92	20.50	25.49
46-55 YEARS	22.53	18.77	25.91	23.90	22.05	26.54
56-65 YEARS	20.85	16.62	25.99	23.15	21.83	25.79
66 OR MORE YEARS	19.66	15.84	22.92	25.00	20.29	25.81

SOURCE: 1ST-4TH QUARTER 1982 AMA SOCIOECONOMIC MONITORING SYSTEM SURVEYS.

*SEE APPENDIX FOR INFORMATION ON DEFINITIONS AND COMPUTATION PROCEDURES.
**EXCLUDES RADIOLOGY, PSYCHIATRY, ANESTHESIOLOGY AND PATHOLOGY, BUT OTHERWISE INCLUDES SPECIALTIES NOT LISTED SEPARATELY.

TABLE 27 (CONTINUED). STANDARD ERROR OF THE MEAN FEE FOR AN OFFICE VISIT WITH AN ESTABLISHED PATIENT (IN DOLLARS), 1982*

| | ALL PHYSICIANS** | GENERAL & FAMILY PRACTICE | SPECIALTY | | | |
			INTERNAL MEDICINE	SURGERY	PEDIATRICS	OBSTETRICS/ GYNECOLOGY
ALL PHYSICIANS	0.15	0.19	0.40	0.28	0.32	0.48
CENSUS DIVISION						
NEW ENGLAND	0.55	0.72	1.25	1.03	0.92	1.79
MIDDLE ATLANTIC	0.44	0.42	1.12	0.81	0.78	1.30
EAST NORTH CENTRAL	0.28	0.36	0.62	0.60	0.59	1.05
WEST NORTH CENTRAL	0.34	0.38	1.18	0.78	1.01	1.02
SOUTH ATLANTIC	0.36	0.37	0.99	0.58	0.68	1.22
EAST SOUTH CENTRAL	0.46	0.45	1.99	0.90	0.74	1.46
WEST SOUTH CENTRAL	0.36	0.40	0.95	0.83	0.92	1.02
MOUNTAIN	0.61	0.81	1.17	1.54	0.95	1.96
PACIFIC	0.40	0.78	1.16	0.81	0.99	0.89
TYPE OF PRACTICE						
SOLO	0.20	0.25	0.56	0.40	0.45	0.67
NON-SOLO	0.21	0.27	0.57	0.41	0.44	0.68
LOCATION						
NONMETROPOLITAN	0.18	0.21	0.40	0.40	0.49	0.57
METROPOLITAN						
LESS THAN 1,000,000	0.23	0.27	0.73	0.43	0.41	0.79
1,000,000 AND OVER	0.60	1.71	1.43	0.96	1.00	1.73
EMPLOYMENT STATUS						
SELF-EMPLOYED	0.16	0.21	0.45	0.32	0.36	0.54
EMPLOYEE	0.33	0.45	0.91	0.65	0.66	1.00
PHYSICIAN AGE						
LESS THAN 36 YEARS	0.36	0.33	0.87	0.99	0.66	1.37
36-45 YEARS	0.26	0.35	0.73	0.49	0.49	0.80
46-55 YEARS	0.32	0.57	0.91	0.51	0.83	1.04
56-65 YEARS	0.30	0.32	0.88	0.64	0.65	1.10
66 OR MORE YEARS	0.42	0.38	1.32	0.97	0.95	1.26

SOURCE: 1ST-4TH QUARTER 1982 AMA SOCIOECONOMIC MONITORING SYSTEM SURVEYS.

*SEE APPENDIX FOR INFORMATION ON DEFINITIONS AND COMPUTATION PROCEDURES.
**EXCLUDES RADIOLOGY, PSYCHIATRY, ANESTHESIOLOGY AND PATHOLOGY, BUT OTHERWISE INCLUDES SPECIALTIES NOT LISTED SEPARATELY.

TABLE 28. MEAN FEE FOR AN OFFICE VISIT WITH AN ESTABLISHED PATIENT (IN DOLLARS), 1973-76, 1978-80, 1982*

	1973	1974	1975	1976	1978	1979	1980	1982**
ALL PHYSICIANS	9.76	10.95	11.76	13.50	15.17	17.17	18.43	21.60
SPECIALTY								
GENERAL/FAMILY PRACTICE	7.52	8.75	9.29	10.65	12.15	13.67	15.18	17.48
INTERNAL MEDICINE	11.28	12.28	13.56	15.52	16.83	19.89	20.46	25.30
SURGERY	10.33	11.27	12.22	13.94	15.91	17.61	19.00	23.57
PEDIATRICS	8.81	10.38	11.07	12.52	13.72	15.65	16.40	21.10
OBSTETRICS/GYNECOLOGY	11.61	13.10	13.73	15.40	18.23	19.04	20.66	25.76
CENSUS DIVISION								
NEW ENGLAND	10.75	11.71	12.57	13.59	15.17	17.60	19.70	22.37
MIDDLE ATLANTIC	11.82	12.60	13.75	15.58	17.41	18.57	20.20	24.17
EAST NORTH CENTRAL	8.87	9.99	10.86	12.26	13.57	15.46	16.69	19.44
WEST NORTH CENTRAL	7.60	9.50	9.00	10.69	11.76	13.55	14.48	16.99
SOUTH ATLANTIC	9.76	11.05	11.79	13.45	15.30	17.54	18.15	21.75
EAST SOUTH CENTRAL	8.47	9.24	9.70	11.34	12.62	15.24	15.52	19.03
WEST SOUTH CENTRAL	8.68	10.17	10.70	12.29	14.33	16.26	16.65	20.78
MOUNTAIN	8.41	9.83	9.92	11.81	13.47	16.35	16.84	21.20
PACIFIC	10.13	11.55	12.94	15.49	17.48	19.53	21.93	25.77
TYPE OF PRACTICE								
SOLO	9.71	10.82	11.69	13.44	15.12	17.23	18.36	21.15
NON-SOLO	9.84	11.13	11.85	13.58	15.26	17.09	18.52	22.10
LOCATION								
NONMETROPOLITAN	6.70	8.05	9.11	9.89	11.07	13.47	13.36	20.76
METROPOLITAN								
LESS THAN 1,000,000	9.01	10.19	10.93	12.35	14.15	15.65	16.67	21.19
1,000,000 AND OVER	11.27	12.38	13.47	15.50	17.14	19.50	21.06	27.89
PHYSICIAN AGE								
LESS THAN 36 YEARS	10.01	10.94	12.46	13.41	15.51	16.94	18.23	21.27
36-45 YEARS	9.73	11.28	11.95	13.92	15.48	17.16	18.98	22.24
46-55 YEARS	9.49	10.90	11.64	13.31	15.11	17.62	18.73	22.53
56-65 YEARS	9.97	10.85	11.42	13.35	15.22	17.15	17.68	20.85
66 OR MORE YEARS	10.06	10.56	11.63	13.30	14.01	16.54	18.08	19.66

SOURCE: 1982, AMA SOCIOECONOMIC MONITORING SYSTEM CORE SURVEYS; 1973-80, AMA PERIODIC SURVEYS OF PHYSICIANS.

*DATA ARE BASED ON INFORMATION FROM PHYSICIANS IN ALL SPECIALTIES EXCLUDING PSYCHIATRY, RADIOLOGY, ANESTHESIOLOGY AND PATHOLOGY. RESULTS FOR YEARS PRIOR TO 1982, OTHER THAN IN THE SPECIALTY BREAKDOWN, MAY DIFFER FROM PREVIOUSLY REPORTED RESULTS BECAUSE OF THE SPECIALTY EXCLUSIONS. SEE APPENDIX FOR INFORMATION ON DEFINITIONS AND COMPUTATION PROCEDURES.
**CAUTION SHOULD BE OBSERVED IN COMPARING 1982 RESULTS WITH RESULTS FOR PREVIOUS YEARS BECAUSE OF CHANGES IN METHODOLOGY MADE IN THE TRANSITION FROM THE PERIODIC SURVEYS OF PHYSICIANS TO THE SOCIOECONOMIC MONITORING SYSTEM.

TABLE 28 (CONTINUED). STANDARD ERROR OF THE MEAN FEE FOR AN OFFICE VISIT WITH AN ESTABLISHED PATIENT (IN DOLLARS), 1973-76, 1978-80, 1982*

	1973	1974	1975	1976	1978	1979	1980	1982**
ALL PHYSICIANS	0.08	0.08	0.09	0.13	0.12	0.15	0.14	0.15
SPECIALTY								
GENERAL/FAMILY PRACTICE	0.07	0.11	0.11	0.09	0.12	0.13	0.14	0.19
INTERNAL MEDICINE	0.19	0.17	0.18	0.47	0.24	0.51	0.25	0.40
SURGERY	0.15	0.14	0.16	0.18	0.23	0.24	0.33	0.28
PEDIATRICS	0.17	0.20	0.20	0.29	0.23	0.27	0.20	0.32
OBSTETRICS/GYNECOLOGY	0.27	0.28	0.38	0.31	0.44	0.41	0.54	0.48
CENSUS DIVISION								
NEW ENGLAND	0.26	0.24	0.32	0.33	0.33	0.48	0.55	0.55
MIDDLE ATLANTIC	0.22	0.21	0.24	0.29	0.38	0.33	0.32	0.44
EAST NORTH CENTRAL	0.14	0.17	0.21	0.18	0.18	0.23	0.24	0.28
WEST NORTH CENTRAL	0.22	0.33	0.22	0.30	0.30	0.33	0.27	0.34
SOUTH ATLANTIC	0.18	0.21	0.17	0.22	0.26	0.64	0.25	0.36
EAST SOUTH CENTRAL	0.34	0.22	0.45	0.26	0.35	0.39	0.35	0.46
WEST SOUTH CENTRAL	0.25	0.26	0.23	0.32	0.35	0.39	0.27	0.36
MOUNTAIN	0.23	0.30	0.23	0.27	0.49	0.54	0.42	0.61
PACIFIC	0.14	0.17	0.22	0.59	0.29	0.34	0.53	0.40
TYPE OF PRACTICE								
SOLO	0.10	0.10	0.13	0.14	0.16	0.24	0.17	0.20
NON-SOLO	0.12	0.12	0.12	0.23	0.17	0.17	0.22	0.21
LOCATION								
NONMETROPOLITAN	0.10	0.20	0.17	0.17	0.25	0.83	0.16	0.18
METROPOLITAN								
LESS THAN 1,000,000	0.10	0.10	0.12	0.11	0.14	0.15	0.13	0.23
1,000,000 AND OVER	0.12	0.12	0.14	0.25	0.19	0.21	0.25	0.60
PHYSICIAN AGE								
LESS THAN 36 YEARS	0.31	0.28	0.35	0.40	0.30	0.41	0.32	0.36
36-45 YEARS	0.13	0.16	0.15	0.34	0.22	0.24	0.24	0.26
46-55 YEARS	0.13	0.14	0.14	0.16	0.21	0.24	0.25	0.32
56-65 YEARS	0.18	0.15	0.18	0.21	0.27	0.26	0.23	0.30
66 OR MORE YEARS	0.26	0.25	0.33	0.36	0.39	0.69	0.72	0.42

SOURCE: 1982, AMA SOCIOECONOMIC MONITORING SYSTEM CORE SURVEYS; 1973-80, AMA PERIODIC SURVEYS OF PHYSICIANS.

*DATA ARE BASED ON INFORMATION FROM PHYSICIANS IN ALL SPECIALTIES EXCLUDING PSYCHIATRY, RADIOLOGY, ANESTHESIOLOGY AND PATHOLOGY. RESULTS FOR YEARS PRIOR TO 1982, OTHER THAN IN THE SPECIALTY BREAKDOWN, MAY DIFFER FROM PREVIOUSLY REPORTED RESULTS BECAUSE OF THE SPECIALTY EXCLUSIONS. SEE APPENDIX FOR INFORMATION ON DEFINITIONS AND COMPUTATION PROCEDURES. **CAUTION SHOULD BE OBSERVED IN COMPARING 1982 RESULTS WITH RESULTS FOR PREVIOUS YEARS BECAUSE OF CHANGES IN METHODOLOGY MADE IN THE TRANSITION FROM THE PERIODIC SURVEYS OF PHYSICIANS TO THE SOCIOECONOMIC MONITORING SYSTEM.

TABLE 29. MEAN FEE FOR AN OFFICE VISIT WITH A NEW PATIENT (IN DOLLARS), 1982*

SPECIALTY

	ALL PHYSICIANS**	GENERAL & FAMILY PRACTICE	INTERNAL MEDICINE	SURGERY	PEDIATRICS	OBSTETRICS/ GYNECOLOGY
ALL PHYSICIANS	38.90	26.58	59.04	39.84	29.63	44.35
CENSUS DIVISION						
NEW ENGLAND	37.00	26.39	53.27	37.51	22.90	38.40
MIDDLE ATLANTIC	45.20	24.93	67.18	45.57	31.55	43.73
EAST NORTH CENTRAL	36.14	24.26	50.17	36.54	26.30	52.37
WEST NORTH CENTRAL	30.41	21.97	36.33	35.26	28.21	38.27
SOUTH ATLANTIC	39.28	26.16	61.10	36.57	29.19	47.83
EAST SOUTH CENTRAL	33.42	26.02	52.44	33.34	33.81	38.23
WEST SOUTH CENTRAL	36.25	24.65	67.34	37.74	27.21	36.82
MOUNTAIN	34.12	26.15	61.50	34.75	29.93	34.74
PACIFIC	46.87	35.87	65.09	51.87	33.54	49.59
TYPE OF PRACTICE						
SOLO	37.88	26.65	55.69	39.28	28.28	47.31
NON-SOLO	39.91	26.47	62.05	40.36	30.64	42.14
LOCATION						
NONMETROPOLITAN	37.27	25.42	55.19	39.58	27.79	46.70
METROPOLITAN						
LESS THAN 1,000,000	37.53	26.98	61.21	36.83	30.00	40.70
1,000,000 AND OVER	51.90	35.87	67.18	53.89	35.44	47.34
EMPLOYMENT STATUS						
SELF-EMPLOYED	38.12	26.46	57.70	39.22	28.44	43.94
EMPLOYEE	41.71	27.23	62.41	42.46	32.52	45.65
PHYSICIAN AGE						
LESS THAN 36 YEARS	38.09	25.94	50.95	41.43	32.79	43.91
36-45 YEARS	39.55	29.64	63.22	39.42	27.63	40.88
46-55 YEARS	39.18	26.20	55.94	40.30	31.05	42.35
56-65 YEARS	38.06	25.20	61.48	39.23	30.27	51.71
66 OR MORE YEARS	38.74	24.83	69.39	39.62	25.11	44.57

SOURCE: 1ST-4TH QUARTER 1982 AMA SOCIOECONOMIC MONITORING SYSTEM SURVEYS.

*SEE APPENDIX FOR INFORMATION ON DEFINITIONS AND COMPUTATION PROCEDURES.
**EXCLUDES RADIOLOGY, PSYCHIATRY, ANESTHESIOLOGY AND PATHOLOGY, BUT OTHERWISE INCLUDES SPECIALTIES NOT LISTED SEPARATELY.

TABLE 29 (CONTINUED). STANDARD ERROR OF THE MEAN FEE FOR AN OFFICE VISIT WITH A NEW PATIENT (IN DOLLARS), 1982*

			SPECIALTY			
	ALL PHYSICIANS**	GENERAL & FAMILY PRACTICE	INTERNAL MEDICINE	SURGERY	PEDIATRICS	OBSTETRICS/ GYNECOLOGY
ALL PHYSICIANS	0.42	0.51	1.41	0.56	0.95	1.33
CENSUS DIVISION						
NEW ENGLAND	1.46	3.12	4.78	1.83	2.08	2.51
MIDDLE ATLANTIC	1.20	1.23	3.74	1.69	2.52	1.69
EAST NORTH CENTRAL	0.97	0.63	2.15	1.22	2.11	7.01
WEST NORTH CENTRAL	1.17	1.98	3.82	1.94	3.10	3.77
SOUTH ATLANTIC	1.00	1.99	2.75	0.97	2.26	3.20
EAST SOUTH CENTRAL	1.10	1.26	4.25	1.20	6.94	1.97
WEST SOUTH CENTRAL	1.43	0.76	7.03	1.51	1.37	1.81
MOUNTAIN	1.20	0.97	4.35	1.87	3.65	1.65
PACIFIC	1.14	1.47	3.59	1.75	1.64	2.41
TYPE OF PRACTICE						
SOLO	0.56	0.71	1.76	0.75	0.85	2.38
NON-SOLO	0.62	0.69	2.19	0.83	1.55	1.41
LOCATION						
NONMETROPOLITAN	0.56	0.53	2.04	0.73	1.15	2.35
METROPOLITAN						
LESS THAN 1,000,000	0.60	1.04	1.85	0.78	1.74	1.70
1,000,000 AND OVER	1.66	2.92	4.47	2.43	2.90	2.10
EMPLOYMENT STATUS						
SELF-EMPLOYED	0.43	0.56	1.36	0.59	0.73	1.48
EMPLOYEE	1.15	1.17	3.90	1.52	2.93	3.00
PHYSICIAN AGE						
LESS THAN 36 YEARS	1.12	0.80	3.31	2.38	3.08	1.97
36-45 YEARS	0.67	1.63	1.92	0.89	1.08	1.10
46-55 YEARS	0.80	1.04	2.25	1.11	2.66	2.80
56-65 YEARS	0.96	0.63	3.29	1.19	1.64	4.60
66 OR MORE YEARS	1.93	1.20	10.95	1.70	1.32	3.23

SOURCE: 1ST-4TH QUARTER 1982 AMA SOCIOECONOMIC MONITORING SYSTEM SURVEYS.

*SEE APPENDIX FOR INFORMATION ON DEFINITIONS AND COMPUTATION PROCEDURES.
**EXCLUDES RADIOLOGY, PSYCHIATRY, ANESTHESIOLOGY AND PATHOLOGY, BUT OTHERWISE INCLUDES SPECIALTIES NOT LISTED SEPARATELY.

TABLE 30. MEAN FEE FOR AN OFFICE VISIT WITH A NEW PATIENT (IN DOLLARS), 1973-76, 1978-80, 1982*

	1973	1974	1975	1976	1978	1979	1980	1982**
ALL PHYSICIANS	15.91	17.88	19.67	22.81	24.93	28.26	30.80	38.90
SPECIALTY								
GENERAL/FAMILY PRACTICE	10.77	12.02	13.11	14.80	16.55	18.21	20.43	26.58
INTERNAL MEDICINE	20.68	23.11	26.11	31.27	32.53	38.18	40.18	59.04
SURGERY	17.62	18.88	20.81	23.29	26.52	29.04	31.83	39.84
PEDIATRICS	12.17	14.48	16.18	17.45	19.03	21.06	22.15	29.63
OBSTETRICS/GYNECOLOGY	19.73	22.08	23.57	27.41	29.85	30.70	34.03	44.35
CENSUS DIVISION								
NEW ENGLAND	16.18	17.95	18.28	20.79	23.27	27.47	31.16	37.00
MIDDLE ATLANTIC	18.76	19.85	22.11	25.49	28.04	30.35	33.10	45.20
EAST NORTH CENTRAL	14.60	15.69	18.13	20.19	22.57	25.64	26.95	36.14
WEST NORTH CENTRAL	12.07	16.09	15.80	19.23	19.09	21.57	23.19	30.41
SOUTH ATLANTIC	16.11	18.76	20.37	23.70	25.18	28.77	30.87	39.28
EAST SOUTH CENTRAL	14.62	15.65	17.29	20.19	21.67	25.35	25.42	33.42
WEST SOUTH CENTRAL	14.20	17.55	19.10	21.87	25.00	27.80	28.25	36.25
MOUNTAIN	13.89	16.53	17.56	21.34	21.36	25.30	28.99	34.12
PACIFIC	17.14	19.14	21.92	25.77	29.04	33.04	38.47	46.87
TYPE OF PRACTICE								
SOLO	15.58	17.48	18.92	21.91	24.43	27.96	29.97	37.88
NON-SOLO	16.40	18.45	20.59	23.90	25.70	28.62	31.78	39.91
LOCATION								
NONMETROPOLITAN	10.65	11.87	14.18	15.64	16.55	19.03	19.22	37.27
METROPOLITAN								
LESS THAN 1,000,000	14.73	17.14	18.53	21.63	23.61	26.23	27.75	37.53
1,000,000 AND OVER	18.42	20.13	22.68	25.78	28.28	32.47	35.95	51.90
PHYSICIAN AGE								
LESS THAN 36 YEARS	16.96	20.01	20.23	23.72	27.76	28.49	31.20	38.09
36-45 YEARS	16.21	18.82	20.71	23.90	26.85	29.99	32.28	39.55
46-55 YEARS	15.56	17.34	19.32	22.30	23.74	28.84	31.79	39.18
56-65 YEARS	15.82	17.88	19.24	22.41	23.97	27.35	28.46	38.06
66 OR MORE YEARS	15.59	16.25	18.38	21.49	21.42	25.26	28.89	38.74

SOURCE: 1982, AMA SOCIOECONOMIC MONITORING SYSTEM CORE SURVEYS; 1973-80, AMA PERIODIC SURVEYS OF PHYSICIANS.

*DATA ARE BASED ON INFORMATION FROM PHYSICIANS IN ALL SPECIALTIES EXCLUDING PSYCHIATRY, RADIOLOGY, ANESTHESIOLOGY AND PATHOLOGY. RESULTS FOR YEARS PRIOR TO 1982, OTHER THAN IN THE SPECIALTY BREAKDOWN, MAY DIFFER FROM PREVIOUSLY REPORTED RESULTS BECAUSE OF THE SPECIALTY EXCLUSIONS. SEE APPENDIX FOR INFORMATION ON DEFINITIONS AND COMPUTATION PROCEDURES.
**CAUTION SHOULD BE OBSERVED IN COMPARING 1982 RESULTS WITH RESULTS FOR PREVIOUS YEARS BECAUSE OF CHANGES IN METHODOLOGY MADE IN THE TRANSITION FROM THE PERIODIC SURVEYS OF PHYSICIANS TO THE SOCIOECONOMIC MONITORING SYSTEM.

TABLE 30 (CONTINUED). STANDARD ERROR OF THE MEAN FEE FOR AN OFFICE VISIT WITH A NEW PATIENT, 1973-76, 1978-80, 1982*

	1973	1974	1975	1976	1978	1979	1980	1982**
ALL PHYSICIANS	0.16	0.19	0.20	0.26	0.29	0.33	0.33	0.42
SPECIALTY								
GENERAL/FAMILY PRACTICE	0.17	0.18	0.19	0.25	0.28	0.28	0.26	0.51
INTERNAL MEDICINE	0.46	0.58	0.62	0.84	0.85	0.99	0.95	1.41
SURGERY	0.28	0.28	0.33	0.39	0.47	0.51	0.54	0.56
PEDIATRICS	0.37	0.55	0.64	0.59	0.54	0.61	0.49	0.95
OBSTETRICS/GYNECOLOGY	0.42	0.43	0.47	0.58	0.67	0.58	0.75	1.33
CENSUS DIVISION								
NEW ENGLAND	0.53	0.63	0.58	0.74	0.81	1.19	1.25	1.46
MIDDLE ATLANTIC	0.42	0.48	0.56	0.66	0.83	0.79	0.81	1.20
EAST NORTH CENTRAL	0.33	0.37	0.47	0.53	0.56	0.77	0.60	0.97
WEST NORTH CENTRAL	0.43	0.65	0.64	0.99	0.91	0.95	0.91	1.17
SOUTH ATLANTIC	0.41	0.55	0.54	0.69	0.70	0.94	0.71	1.00
EAST SOUTH CENTRAL	0.68	0.86	0.74	1.08	1.13	1.09	0.96	1.10
WEST SOUTH CENTRAL	0.52	0.70	0.73	0.89	1.14	1.10	1.40	1.43
MOUNTAIN	0.62	0.86	0.79	1.14	0.90	1.04	1.45	1.20
PACIFIC	0.38	0.40	0.49	0.66	0.71	0.86	0.94	1.14
TYPE OF PRACTICE								
SOLO	0.20	0.24	0.26	0.34	0.36	0.46	0.42	0.56
NON-SOLO	0.26	0.29	0.31	0.39	0.47	0.47	0.52	0.62
LOCATION								
NONMETROPOLITAN	0.28	0.33	0.36	0.58	0.55	0.91	0.42	0.56
METROPOLITAN								
LESS THAN 1,000,000	0.21	0.28	0.28	0.36	0.38	0.42	0.40	0.60
1,000,000 AND OVER	0.26	0.29	0.34	0.41	0.47	0.53	0.55	1.66
PHYSICIAN AGE								
LESS THAN 36 YEARS	0.66	0.88	0.67	1.04	0.91	1.09	0.97	1.12
36-45 YEARS	0.29	0.38	0.38	0.50	0.59	0.63	0.59	0.67
46-55 YEARS	0.29	0.32	0.37	0.44	0.46	0.61	0.75	0.80
56-65 YEARS	0.33	0.38	0.43	0.53	0.64	0.65	0.58	0.96
66 OR MORE YEARS	0.47	0.49	0.60	0.84	0.69	0.97	0.94	1.93

SOURCE: 1982, AMA SOCIOECONOMIC MONITORING SYSTEM CORE SURVEYS; 1973-80, AMA PERIODIC SURVEYS OF PHYSICIANS.

*DATA ARE BASED ON INFORMATION FROM PHYSICIANS IN ALL SPECIALTIES EXCLUDING PSYCHIATRY, RADIOLOGY, ANESTHESIOLOGY AND PATHOLOGY. RESULTS FOR YEARS PRIOR TO 1982, OTHER THAN IN THE SPECIALTY BREAKDOWN, MAY DIFFER FROM PREVIOUSLY REPORTED RESULTS BECAUSE OF THE SPECIALTY EXCLUSIONS. SEE APPENDIX FOR INFORMATION ON DEFINITIONS AND COMPUTATION PROCEDURES.
**CAUTION SHOULD BE OBSERVED IN COMPARING 1982 RESULTS WITH RESULTS FOR PREVIOUS YEARS BECAUSE OF CHANGES IN METHODOLOGY MADE IN THE TRANSITION FROM THE PERIODIC SURVEYS OF PHYSICIANS TO THE SOCIOECONOMIC MONITORING SYSTEM.

TABLE 31.   MEAN FEE FOR A FOLLOW-UP HOSPITAL VISIT (IN DOLLARS), 1982*

	ALL PHYSICIANS**	SPECIALTY				
		GENERAL & FAMILY PRACTICE	INTERNAL MEDICINE	SURGERY	PEDIATRICS	OBSTETRICS/ GYNECOLOGY
ALL PHYSICIANS	24.73	21.18	27.02	24.83	24.01	26.12
CENSUS DIVISION						
NEW ENGLAND	23.55	20.09	25.07	24.65	19.33	
MIDDLE ATLANTIC	28.41	23.10	30.26	31.91	24.46	25.01
EAST NORTH CENTRAL	23.45	20.95	24.75	25.21	21.90	25.89
WEST NORTH CENTRAL	21.18	16.95	23.05	25.15	22.49	17.45
SOUTH ATLANTIC	25.15	20.78	27.97	22.50	25.15	34.31
EAST SOUTH CENTRAL	20.43	19.09	22.94	18.66	17.95	19.18
WEST SOUTH CENTRAL	23.81	21.99	26.03	22.01	24.33	25.09
MOUNTAIN	24.34	22.24	26.50	21.84	24.55	
PACIFIC	30.90	28.89	32.53	30.36	31.28	24.20
TYPE OF PRACTICE						
SOLO	24.85	21.53	27.73	24.06	24.78	24.22
NON-SOLO	24.62	20.72	26.45	25.36	23.53	27.67
LOCATION						
NONMETROPOLITAN	24.38	20.82	27.38	24.40	24.64	26.91
METROPOLITAN						
LESS THAN 1,000,000	23.14	20.66	24.85	22.21	22.53	24.44
1,000,000 AND OVER	32.06	27.70	32.36	35.65	29.22	28.45
EMPLOYMENT STATUS						
SELF-EMPLOYED	24.23	21.32	26.82	22.91	24.18	24.75
EMPLOYEE	26.51	20.17	27.58	30.89	23.52	30.63
PHYSICIAN AGE						
LESS THAN 36 YEARS	24.65	20.30	26.59	24.99	22.20	31.82
36-45 YEARS	25.94	22.49	27.25	25.99	25.38	21.70
46-55 YEARS	24.91	22.52	26.44	25.33	24.33	28.39
56-65 YEARS	23.35	19.77	28.26	21.31	24.37	25.17
66 OR MORE YEARS	22.11	20.36	25.42	25.57	17.33	27.78

SOURCE: 1ST-4TH QUARTER 1982 AMA SOCIOECONOMIC MONITORING SYSTEM SURVEYS.

*SEE APPENDIX FOR INFORMATION ON DEFINITIONS AND COMPUTATION PROCEDURES.
**EXCLUDES RADIOLOGY, PSYCHIATRY, ANESTHESIOLOGY AND PATHOLOGY, BUT OTHERWISE INCLUDES SPECIALTIES NOT LISTED SEPARATELY.

TABLE 31 (CONTINUED). STANDARD ERROR OF THE MEAN FEE FOR A FOLLOW-UP HOSPITAL VISIT (IN DOLLARS), 1982*

	ALL PHYSICIANS**	SPECIALTY				
		GENERAL & FAMILY PRACTICE	INTERNAL MEDICINE	SURGERY	PEDIATRICS	OBSTETRICS/ GYNECOLOGY
ALL PHYSICIANS	0.23	0.36	0.46	0.52	0.55	0.97
CENSUS DIVISION						
NEW ENGLAND	0.59	1.01	0.87	1.37	1.25	
MIDDLE ATLANTIC	0.70	1.27	1.10	1.93	1.51	1.59
EAST NORTH CENTRAL	0.46	0.72	0.87	1.27	0.95	1.36
WEST NORTH CENTRAL	0.74	0.84	1.72	1.85	2.32	2.14
SOUTH ATLANTIC	0.71	1.05	1.51	1.21	1.52	3.10
EAST SOUTH CENTRAL	0.51	0.75	1.33	0.85	1.25	1.52
WEST SOUTH CENTRAL	0.48	0.87	0.92	0.90	1.50	2.03
MOUNTAIN	1.05	2.02	2.51	1.27	1.95	
PACIFIC	0.58	1.23	1.17	1.28	1.30	1.36
TYPE OF PRACTICE						
SOLO	0.34	0.50	0.78	0.66	0.79	0.96
NON-SOLO	0.30	0.51	0.53	0.77	0.76	1.56
LOCATION						
NONMETROPOLITAN	0.32	0.46	0.73	0.61	0.79	1.22
METROPOLITAN						
LESS THAN 1,000,000	0.31	0.55	0.62	0.63	0.81	1.80
1,000,000 AND OVER	0.85	1.53	1.15	2.68	2.00	1.24
EMPLOYMENT STATUS						
SELF-EMPLOYED	0.24	0.39	0.54	0.46	0.60	1.08
EMPLOYEE	0.57	0.99	0.90	1.62	1.31	2.04
PHYSICIAN AGE						
LESS THAN 36 YEARS	0.53	0.74	0.91	1.56	1.62	2.62
36-45 YEARS	0.36	0.85	0.57	0.92	0.87	1.01
46-55 YEARS	0.49	0.81	1.02	1.07	1.11	2.41
56-65 YEARS	0.59	0.64	1.81	0.83	1.19	1.39
66 OR MORE YEARS	0.75	0.99	1.97	1.42	1.26	3.50

SOURCE: 1ST-4TH QUARTER 1982 AMA SOCIOECONOMIC MONITORING SYSTEM SURVEYS.

*SEE APPENDIX FOR INFORMATION ON DEFINITIONS AND COMPUTATION PROCEDURES.
**EXCLUDES RADIOLOGY, PSYCHIATRY, ANESTHESIOLOGY AND PATHOLOGY, BUT OTHERWISE INCLUDES SPECIALTIES NOT LISTED SEPARATELY.

TABLE 32. MEAN FEE FOR A FOLLOW-UP HOSPITAL VISIT (IN DOLLARS), 1973-76, 1978-80, 1982*

	1973	1974	1975	1976	1978	1979	1980	1982**
ALL PHYSICIANS	13.46	15.52	16.98	19.92	22.28	24.06	26.70	24.73
SPECIALTY								
GENERAL/FAMILY PRACTICE	10.53	12.79	13.51	16.11	17.89	19.06	21.84	21.18
INTERNAL MEDICINE	14.65	16.47	18.56	21.02	23.95	25.11	27.93	27.02
SURGERY	15.30	16.65	18.29	20.95	23.71	24.91	28.92	24.83
PEDIATRICS	12.19	13.91	16.14	18.59	20.30	23.32	22.61	24.01
OBSTETRICS/GYNECOLOGY	14.19	16.96	17.99	23.25	24.79	27.03	27.69	26.12
CENSUS DIVISION								
NEW ENGLAND	13.39	15.28	15.56	20.88	19.71	23.04	26.07	23.55
MIDDLE ATLANTIC	16.27	17.80	19.26	22.79	25.43	27.29	29.19	28.41
EAST NORTH CENTRAL	12.01	13.77	15.94	18.11	20.33	21.19	24.02	23.45
WEST NORTH CENTRAL	10.94	12.98	13.41	15.74	17.58	18.79	21.09	21.18
SOUTH ATLANTIC	13.60	15.74	17.11	20.09	23.43	25.53	27.05	25.15
EAST SOUTH CENTRAL	11.21	13.98	14.61	15.46	18.82	19.65	21.23	20.43
WEST SOUTH CENTRAL	12.23	14.90	16.10	18.71	20.26	24.36	24.48	23.81
MOUNTAIN	12.82	14.75	15.29	18.31	19.06	22.16	23.91	24.34
PACIFIC	14.68	17.24	19.56	22.78	26.23	26.57	32.57	30.90
TYPE OF PRACTICE								
SOLO	13.51	15.69	17.08	20.09	22.52	24.23	26.79	24.85
NON-SOLO	13.39	15.29	16.86	19.73	21.91	23.86	26.60	24.62
LOCATION								
NONMETROPOLITAN	9.74	11.29	12.78	15.00	16.92	17.65	19.54	24.38
METROPOLITAN								
LESS THAN 1,000,000	12.59	14.62	15.91	18.63	20.53	22.19	24.00	23.14
1,000,000 AND OVER	15.37	17.54	19.49	22.43	25.29	27.49	30.66	32.06
PHYSICIAN AGE								
LESS THAN 36 YEARS	13.11	17.07	17.60	19.23	23.78	23.90	28.00	24.65
36-45 YEARS	13.39	15.79	17.14	20.52	23.44	25.03	26.64	25.94
46-55 YEARS	13.68	15.02	16.86	20.13	21.25	24.92	26.69	24.91
56-65 YEARS	13.66	15.86	17.00	19.10	21.71	22.97	26.84	23.35
66 OR MORE YEARS	12.82	14.59	16.23	19.88	20.98	22.04	24.82	22.11

SOURCE: 1982, AMA SOCIOECONOMIC MONITORING SYSTEM CORE SURVEYS; 1973-80, AMA PERIODIC SURVEYS OF PHYSICIANS.

*DATA ARE BASED ON INFORMATION FROM PHYSICIANS IN ALL SPECIALTIES EXCLUDING PSYCHIATRY, RADIOLOGY, ANESTHESIOLOGY AND PATHOLOGY. RESULTS FOR YEARS PRIOR TO 1982, OTHER THAN IN THE SPECIALTY BREAKDOWN, MAY DIFFER FROM PREVIOUSLY REPORTED RESULTS BECAUSE OF THE SPECIALTY EXCLUSIONS. SEE APPENDIX FOR INFORMATION ON DEFINITIONS AND COMPUTATION PROCEDURES.

**CAUTION SHOULD BE OBSERVED IN COMPARING 1982 RESULTS WITH RESULTS FOR PREVIOUS YEARS BECAUSE OF CHANGES IN METHODOLOGY MADE IN THE TRANSITION FROM THE PERIODIC SURVEYS OF PHYSICIANS TO THE SOCIOECONOMIC MONITORING SYSTEM.

TABLE 32 (CONTINUED). STANDARD ERROR OF THE MEAN FEE FOR A FOLLOW-UP HOSPITAL VISIT (IN DOLLARS), 1973-76, 1978-80, 1982*

	1973	1974	1975	1976	1978	1979	1980	1982**
ALL PHYSICIANS	0.17	0.18	0.20	0.27	0.26	0.28	0.41	0.23
SPECIALTY								
GENERAL/FAMILY PRACTICE	0.21	0.27	0.27	0.34	0.39	0.39	0.91	0.36
INTERNAL MEDICINE	0.38	0.39	0.46	0.61	0.60	0.59	0.61	0.46
SURGERY	0.35	0.37	0.40	0.58	0.53	0.55	0.92	0.52
PEDIATRICS	0.38	0.54	0.63	0.68	0.69	0.84	0.75	0.55
OBSTETRICS/GYNECOLOGY	0.58	0.64	0.62	0.90	0.87	0.90	0.94	0.97
CENSUS DIVISION								
NEW ENGLAND	0.57	0.70	0.64	1.84	0.83	0.94	1.32	0.59
MIDDLE ATLANTIC	0.45	0.48	0.56	0.65	0.75	0.75	1.43	0.70
EAST NORTH CENTRAL	0.33	0.36	0.43	0.52	0.55	0.61	0.60	0.46
WEST NORTH CENTRAL	0.53	0.55	0.54	0.67	0.74	0.81	0.90	0.74
SOUTH ATLANTIC	0.44	0.48	0.50	0.57	0.70	0.78	0.77	0.71
EAST SOUTH CENTRAL	0.71	0.76	1.04	0.70	0.91	0.91	0.84	0.51
WEST SOUTH CENTRAL	0.49	0.62	0.58	0.68	0.71	0.93	0.81	0.48
MOUNTAIN	0.73	0.93	0.72	1.09	0.80	0.88	1.06	1.05
PACIFIC	0.41	0.47	0.52	0.80	0.72	0.70	1.37	0.58
TYPE OF PRACTICE								
SOLO	0.22	0.25	0.27	0.38	0.35	0.40	0.57	0.34
NON-SOLO	0.26	0.27	0.29	0.38	0.39	0.39	0.58	0.30
LOCATION								
NONMETROPOLITAN	0.33	0.36	0.36	0.53	0.60	0.52	0.58	0.32
METROPOLITAN								
LESS THAN 1,000,000	0.24	0.27	0.29	0.41	0.35	0.39	0.38	0.31
1,000,000 AND OVER	0.26	0.29	0.32	0.41	0.43	0.45	0.76	0.85
PHYSICIAN AGE								
LESS THAN 36 YEARS	0.62	0.87	0.64	0.81	0.77	0.97	1.07	0.53
36-45 YEARS	0.30	0.36	0.36	0.53	0.54	0.56	0.51	0.36
46-55 YEARS	0.30	0.31	0.36	0.44	0.43	0.55	0.58	0.49
56-65 YEARS	0.36	0.38	0.44	0.46	0.55	0.54	1.44	0.59
66 OR MORE YEARS	0.47	0.52	0.57	1.24	0.84	0.66	0.77	0.75

SOURCE: 1982, AMA SOCIOECONOMIC MONITORING SYSTEM CORE SURVEYS; 1973-80, AMA PERIODIC SURVEYS OF PHYSICIANS.

*DATA ARE BASED ON INFORMATION FROM PHYSICIANS IN ALL SPECIALTIES EXCLUDING PSYCHIATRY, RADIOLOGY, ANESTHESIOLOGY AND PATHOLOGY. RESULTS FOR YEARS PRIOR TO 1982, OTHER THAN IN THE SPECIALTY BREAKDOWN, MAY DIFFER FROM PREVIOUSLY REPORTED RESULTS BECAUSE OF THE SPECIALTY EXCLUSIONS. SEE APPENDIX FOR INFORMATION ON DEFINITIONS AND COMPUTATION PROCEDURES.
**CAUTION SHOULD BE OBSERVED IN COMPARING 1982 RESULTS WITH RESULTS FOR PREVIOUS YEARS BECAUSE OF CHANGES IN METHODOLOGY MADE IN THE TRANSITION FROM THE PERIODIC SURVEYS OF PHYSICIANS TO THE SOCIOECONOMIC MONITORING SYSTEM.

TABLE 33. MEAN PROFESSIONAL EXPENSES OF SELF-EMPLOYED PHYSICIANS (IN THOUSANDS OF DOLLARS), 1982*

	ALL PHYSICIANS**	SPECIALTY								
		GP/FP	INT MED	SURG	PED	OB/GYN	RAD	PSYCH	ANES	PATH
ALL PHYSICIANS	78.4	75.7	75.8	105.0	66.7	109.0	68.1	37.2	52.3	81.9
CENSUS DIVISION										
NEW ENGLAND	69.6	52.0	74.1	82.9	46.8	84.5	26.6	23.1	.	.
MIDDLE ATLANTIC	59.0	44.8	59.9	83.5	58.7	105.4	45.9	48.0	.	.
EAST NORTH CENTRAL	71.2	72.0	74.6	98.2	.	.	.	39.4	41.0	.
WEST NORTH CENTRAL	87.8	82.1	93.1	111.6	63.1	121.7	69.3	.	.	.
SOUTH ATLANTIC	82.3	70.9	70.8	112.7	.	.	.	35.7	.	.
EAST SOUTH CENTRAL	86.3	80.4	83.7	119.8	.	.	.	.	.	.
WEST SOUTH CENTRAL	100.7	94.8	106.4	116.9	120.8	114.5	89.7	29.8	48.4	.
MOUNTAIN	77.6	78.2	62.9	95.4	.	.	.	.	.	.
PACIFIC	78.1	85.5	75.2	111.8	50.4	104.0	76.9	32.0	41.1	.
TYPE OF PRACTICE										
SOLO	71.2	65.4	72.3	95.2	60.7	101.0	69.3	38.1	42.4	33.0
NON-SOLO	87.9	92.4	80.9	120.3	72.2	119.6	67.8	33.2	59.5	96.5
LOCATION										
NONMETROPOLITAN	80.0	78.2	77.9	102.9	66.8	112.5	73.3	34.6	43.3	92.9
METROPOLITAN										
LESS THAN 1,000,000	77.4	67.3	71.4	108.0	71.2	109.2	58.8	41.0	62.0	75.4
1,000,000 AND OVER	74.5	94.1	79.2	104.0	50.8	85.2	76.3	38.2	.	.
PHYSICIAN AGE										
LESS THAN 36 YEARS	55.6	60.0	49.5	82.4	74.9	.	.	26.5	39.6	.
36-45 YEARS	77.6	88.2	75.3	108.3	59.9	99.7	72.5	27.7	46.4	27.9
46-55 YEARS	96.4	95.8	92.2	113.0	75.3	144.3	84.1	42.7	85.2	140.9
56-65 YEARS	80.4	74.6	79.6	112.5	64.1	108.2	44.6	49.4	38.5	70.7
66 OR MORE YEARS	56.0	50.5	78.8	61.6	.	46.6	.	31.2	.	.

SOURCE: 1983 AMA SOCIOECONOMIC MONITORING SYSTEM CORE SURVEY.

*SEE APPENDIX FOR INFORMATION ON DEFINITIONS AND COMPUTATION PROCEDURES.
**INCLUDES PHYSICIANS IN SPECIALTIES NOT LISTED SEPARATELY.
. INDICATES FEWER THAN TEN OBSERVATIONS.

TABLE 33 (CONTINUED). STANDARD ERROR OF MEAN PROFESSIONAL EXPENSES OF SELF-EMPLOYED PHYSICIANS (IN THOUSANDS OF DOLLARS), 1982*

	ALL PHYSICIANS**	SPECIALTY								
		GP/FP	INT MED	SURG	PED	OB/GYN	RAD	PSYCH	ANES	PATH
ALL PHYSICIANS	1.84	2.90	3.48	5.00	4.75	6.33	10.38	3.84	6.31	21.17
CENSUS DIVISION										
NEW ENGLAND	7.98	9.49	10.73	10.27	7.85	9.80	10.72	4.79	.	.
MIDDLE ATLANTIC	4.13	5.07	9.85	10.48	7.39	10.72	11.05	15.75	.	.
EAST NORTH CENTRAL	3.58	6.10	7.06	10.92	.	.	.	5.79	6.82	.
WEST NORTH CENTRAL	8.82	10.66	23.62	24.38	.	.	.	.	.	.
SOUTH ATLANTIC	4.79	5.45	7.23	12.53	8.44	22.02	19.63	6.26	.	.
EAST SOUTH CENTRAL	7.65	8.69	16.42	26.81	.	.	.	.	.	.
WEST SOUTH CENTRAL	5.97	9.64	13.18	10.17	25.31	17.63	29.00	5.38	12.37	.
MOUNTAIN	5.85	11.16	10.12	9.89	.	.	.	.	.	.
PACIFIC	4.65	10.35	7.84	16.08	8.79	10.53	26.00	7.86	8.59	.
TYPE OF PRACTICE										
SOLO	1.92	3.13	4.30	4.73	7.02	6.70	18.02	4.55	5.05	6.92
NON-SOLO	3.40	5.38	5.80	10.35	6.42	11.74	11.95	4.39	10.19	27.00
LOCATION										
NONMETROPOLITAN	2.52	3.84	5.26	5.80	7.00	9.53	17.31	6.36	7.04	34.35
METROPOLITAN										
LESS THAN 1,000,000	3.01	3.87	4.94	8.47	7.89	9.34	11.84	6.15	10.29	31.33
1,000,000 AND OVER	6.10	18.47	10.03	25.26	8.92	13.81	29.28	5.09	.	.
PHYSICIAN AGE										
LESS THAN 36 YEARS	3.10	5.77	5.93	12.02	10.70	7.27	14.99	4.39	8.39	7.30
36-45 YEARS	3.12	6.25	5.33	9.21	7.24	16.17	23.81	3.16	6.71	.
46-55 YEARS	4.41	7.38	7.84	8.66	13.69	11.31	11.05	5.78	24.34	48.63
56-65 YEARS	4.09	5.81	9.48	11.61	6.79	11.13	.	15.19	8.75	37.49
66 OR MORE YEARS	3.67	4.38	14.11	7.58	.	.	.	6.68	.	.

SOURCE: 1983 AMA SOCIOECONOMIC MONITORING SYSTEM CORE SURVEY.

*SEE APPENDIX FOR INFORMATION ON DEFINITIONS AND COMPUTATION PROCEDURES.
**INCLUDES PHYSICIANS IN SPECIALTIES NOT LISTED SEPARATELY.
. INDICATES FEWER THAN TEN OBSERVATIONS.

TABLE 34. MEAN PROFESSIONAL EXPENSES (IN THOUSANDS OF DOLLARS), 1973-75, 1977-79, 1981-82*

	1973	1974	1975	1977	1978	1979	1981**	1982**
ALL PHYSICIANS	32.2	34.0	38.5	45.5	46.4	52.9	74.0	78.4
SPECIALTY								
GENERAL/FAMILY PRACTICE	34.0	36.7	38.6	46.1	47.8	55.7	72.7	75.7
INTERNAL MEDICINE	34.0	35.8	40.4	45.6	44.8	52.5	76.0	75.8
SURGERY	38.0	39.3	49.1	60.4	63.4	69.3	92.1	105.0
PEDIATRICS	32.4	30.0	34.6	39.1	35.1	51.0	63.9	66.7
OBSTETRICS/GYNECOLOGY	37.2	41.9	48.5	60.9	61.9	67.0	99.6	109.0
RADIOLOGY	35.4	36.4	36.2	43.3	42.1	51.0	94.1	68.1
PSYCHIATRY	14.2	14.0	18.7	19.3	24.2	23.1	28.3	37.2
ANESTHESIOLOGY	14.0	19.3	20.0	25.9	25.3	26.3	48.4	52.3
CENSUS DIVISION								
NEW ENGLAND	26.3	24.6	28.4	36.5	31.1	38.0	53.8	69.6
MIDDLE ATLANTIC	24.6	28.0	33.4	34.2	39.6	41.8	65.7	59.0
EAST NORTH CENTRAL	32.8	33.8	39.9	41.4	45.8	52.1	72.4	71.2
WEST NORTH CENTRAL	34.4	35.4	37.7	45.6	47.4	52.0	78.3	87.8
SOUTH ATLANTIC	32.4	37.1	36.8	48.9	45.8	54.9	78.4	82.3
EAST SOUTH CENTRAL	36.0	40.2	48.0	47.5	53.1	66.0	92.0	86.3
WEST SOUTH CENTRAL	40.2	39.0	44.8	56.4	52.4	61.2	83.3	100.7
MOUNTAIN	33.9	34.2	36.5	52.9	48.7	54.5	62.9	77.6
PACIFIC	36.2	38.4	44.3	53.0	53.1	60.2	77.8	78.1
TYPE OF PRACTICE								
SOLO	29.4	33.2	38.0	43.6	47.7	50.5	71.1	71.2
NON-SOLO	36.6	35.0	39.1	48.6	44.7	55.8	79.7	87.9
LOCATION								
NONMETROPOLITAN	34.6	33.9	40.0	47.5	53.0	62.1	70.6	80.0
METROPOLITAN								
LESS THAN 1,000,000	34.3	35.4	38.7	48.2	49.1	53.4	82.0	77.4
1,000,000 AND OVER	29.9	32.9	38.0	42.8	42.7	50.9	67.1	74.5
PHYSICIAN AGE								
LESS THAN 36 YEARS	21.6	23.3	29.0	31.1	28.2	37.4	51.4	55.6
36-45 YEARS	35.2	36.4	41.3	52.2	47.9	59.6	76.3	77.6
46-55 YEARS	35.6	39.9	43.2	52.1	55.9	63.3	92.3	96.4
56-65 YEARS	31.8	32.6	39.0	43.6	48.3	49.3	67.7	80.4
66 OR MORE YEARS	22.3	23.7	24.2	28.6	32.2	36.4	68.3	56.0

SOURCE: 1981-82, AMA SOCIOECONOMIC MONITORING SYSTEM CORE SURVEYS; 1973-79, AMA PERIODIC SURVEYS OF PHYSICIANS.

*DATA, OTHER THAN IN THE SPECIALTY BREAKDOWN, ARE BASED ON RESPONSES FROM PHYSICIANS IN ALL SPECIALTIES. SEE APPENDIX FOR INFORMATION ON DEFINITIONS AND COMPUTATION PROCEDURES.

**CAUTION SHOULD BE OBSERVED IN COMPARING 1981 AND 1982 RESULTS WITH RESULTS FOR PREVIOUS YEARS BECAUSE OF CHANGES IN METHODOLOGY MADE IN THE TRANSITION FROM THE PERIODIC SURVEYS OF PHYSICIANS TO THE SOCIOECONOMIC MONITORING SYSTEM.

TABLE 34 (CONTINUED). STANDARD ERROR OF MEAN PROFESSIONAL EXPENSES (IN THOUSANDS OF DOLLARS), 1973-75, 1977-79, 1981-82*

	1973	1974	1975	1977	1978	1979	1981**	1982**
ALL PHYSICIANS	0.50	0.47	0.54	0.87	0.87	1.01	2.39	1.84
SPECIALTY								
GENERAL/FAMILY PRACTICE	0.89	0.99	1.04	1.51	1.65	2.09	4.31	2.90
INTERNAL MEDICINE	1.19	1.21	1.25	1.58	1.56	2.17	5.24	3.48
SURGERY	1.05	0.84	1.22	2.19	2.41	2.26	5.56	5.00
PEDIATRICS	1.66	1.35	1.76	2.19	2.14	3.37	9.24	4.75
OBSTETRICS/GYNECOLOGY	1.33	1.82	2.16	3.42	3.29	4.47	11.85	6.33
RADIOLOGY	4.05	3.72	3.78	6.89	5.40	8.22	16.15	10.38
PSYCHIATRY	0.72	0.65	1.05	1.22	1.67	2.35	2.08	3.84
ANESTHESIOLOGY	1.12	1.49	1.27	2.47	2.43	2.56	9.19	6.31
CENSUS DIVISION								
NEW ENGLAND	1.68	1.33	1.71	2.44	2.01	2.60	6.83	7.98
MIDDLE ATLANTIC	0.81	0.87	1.11	1.20	1.73	2.08	4.79	4.13
EAST NORTH CENTRAL	1.28	1.12	1.35	1.52	2.33	2.43	5.98	3.58
WEST NORTH CENTRAL	1.60	1.73	2.15	2.90	3.23	2.89	6.13	8.82
SOUTH ATLANTIC	1.21	1.50	1.30	2.15	1.94	2.45	7.16	4.79
EAST SOUTH CENTRAL	2.53	2.66	3.69	3.10	4.57	6.13	17.53	7.65
WEST SOUTH CENTRAL	2.87	1.53	1.80	4.27	3.35	3.67	6.71	5.97
MOUNTAIN	1.92	1.52	1.82	6.69	2.85	3.67	6.31	5.85
PACIFIC	1.15	1.30	1.45	2.36	2.40	2.83	5.11	4.65
TYPE OF PRACTICE								
SOLO	0.51	0.56	0.68	0.97	1.13	1.05	2.89	1.92
NON-SOLO	0.99	0.78	0.87	1.64	1.36	1.85	4.23	3.40
LOCATION								
NONMETROPOLITAN	1.42	1.16	1.71	2.21	2.47	3.93	2.84	2.52
METROPOLITAN								
LESS THAN 1,000,000	0.90	0.78	0.85	1.57	1.38	1.50	5.18	3.01
1,000,000 AND OVER	0.62	0.67	0.77	1.11	1.25	1.45	4.69	6.10
PHYSICIAN AGE								
LESS THAN 36 YEARS	1.86	1.15	2.06	1.64	2.21	1.76	3.86	3.10
36-45 YEARS	1.11	0.91	1.02	1.72	1.76	2.28	3.95	3.12
46-55 YEARS	0.85	0.93	1.00	1.85	1.96	2.30	6.41	4.41
56-65 YEARS	0.92	0.92	1.16	1.79	1.60	1.61	3.83	4.09
66 OR MORE YEARS	1.07	1.14	1.14	1.61	1.51	2.07	9.01	3.67

SOURCE: 1981-82, AMA SOCIOECONOMIC MONITORING SYSTEM CORE SURVEYS; 1973-79, AMA PERIODIC SURVEYS OF PHYSICIANS.

*DATA, OTHER THAN IN THE SPECIALTY BREAKDOWN, ARE BASED ON RESPONSES FROM PHYSICIANS IN ALL SPECIALTIES. SEE APPENDIX FOR INFORMATION ON DEFINITIONS AND COMPUTATION PROCEDURES.
**CAUTION SHOULD BE OBSERVED IN COMPARING 1981 AND 1982 RESULTS WITH RESULTS FOR PREVIOUS YEARS BECAUSE OF CHANGES IN METHODOLOGY MADE IN THE TRANSITION FROM THE PERIODIC SURVEYS OF PHYSICIANS TO THE SOCIOECONOMIC MONITORING SYSTEM.

TABLE 35. MEDIAN PROFESSIONAL EXPENSES OF SELF-EMPLOYED PHYSICIANS (IN THOUSANDS OF DOLLARS), 1982*

	ALL PHYSICIANS**	SPECIALTY								
		GP/FP	INT MED	SURG	PED	OB/GYN	RAD	PSYCH	ANES	PATH
ALL PHYSICIANS	60.0	64.0	66.0	75.5	57.0	95.0	38.0	28.0	31.5	22.5
CENSUS DIVISION										
NEW ENGLAND	47.0	51.0	62.0	59.0	41.0	78.5	10.0	19.0	.	.
MIDDLE ATLANTIC	47.0	44.0	44.0	65.5	55.0	101.5	41.5	24.0	.	.
EAST NORTH CENTRAL	60.0	62.0	70.0	69.0	.	.	.	30.0	34.0	.
WEST NORTH CENTRAL	64.0	64.0	86.0	77.5	.	.	.	.	.	.
SOUTH ATLANTIC	60.5	61.0	64.0	85.0	52.0	88.0	41.0	33.0	.	.
EAST SOUTH CENTRAL	70.5	67.0	78.0	68.0	.	.	.	.	.	.
WEST SOUTH CENTRAL	80.0	83.5	86.0	91.0	97.0	89.0	43.5	34.0	39.0	.
MOUNTAIN	63.0	74.0	56.5	82.0	.	.	.	.	.	.
PACIFIC	60.0	69.0	66.0	80.0	41.0	99.0	37.0	22.5	33.0	.
TYPE OF PRACTICE										
SOLO	59.0	58.5	64.0	71.0	45.5	89.0	47.5	28.0	32.0	27.0
NON-SOLO	64.0	83.0	73.0	90.0	63.0	107.0	33.0	28.0	31.0	19.0
LOCATION										
NONMETROPOLITAN	60.0	64.0	68.0	74.0	53.5	89.0	41.5	22.5	30.0	18.0
METROPOLITAN										
LESS THAN 1,000,000	62.0	63.0	64.0	81.0	66.0	100.0	30.0	31.0	36.0	22.0
1,000,000 AND OVER	57.0	74.0	75.0	66.5	44.0	79.0	37.0	30.0	.	.
PHYSICIAN AGE										
LESS THAN 36 YEARS	47.0	57.0	38.0	62.5	83.0	89.0	54.0	29.0	25.5	14.5
36-45 YEARS	63.0	78.0	70.0	80.5	44.0	117.0	41.5	23.0	33.0	46.5
46-55 YEARS	69.0	83.0	75.0	96.0	55.0	95.5	31.5	31.5	45.0	26.0
56-65 YEARS	63.0	62.0	65.0	80.0	60.0	39.0	.	31.0	24.0	.
66 OR MORE YEARS	46.0	44.0	70.0	54.0	.	.	.	26.0	.	.

SOURCE: 1983 AMA SOCIOECONOMIC MONITORING SYSTEM CORE SURVEY.

*SEE APPENDIX FOR INFORMATION ON DEFINITIONS AND COMPUTATION PROCEDURES.
**INCLUDES PHYSICIANS IN SPECIALTIES NOT LISTED SEPARATELY.
. INDICATES FEWER THAN TEN OBSERVATIONS.

TABLE 36. MEDIAN PROFESSIONAL EXPENSES (IN THOUSANDS OF DOLLARS), 1973-75, 1977-79, 1981-82*

	1973	1974	1975	1977	1978	1979	1981**	1982**
ALL PHYSICIANS	27.0	30.0	31.0	36.0	35.0	40.0	52.0	60.0
SPECIALTY								
GENERAL/FAMILY PRACTICE	30.0	32.0	35.0	40.0	40.0	44.0	57.5	64.0
INTERNAL MEDICINE	30.0	32.0	35.0	39.0	40.0	42.0	60.0	66.0
SURGERY	32.0	35.0	40.0	47.0	50.0	52.0	70.0	75.5
PEDIATRICS	29.0	27.0	30.0	38.0	31.0	40.0	50.0	57.0
OBSTETRICS/GYNECOLOGY	35.0	37.0	40.0	50.0	50.0	59.5	75.0	95.0
RADIOLOGY	20.0	24.5	20.0	20.0	20.0	20.0	48.0	38.0
PSYCHIATRY	11.0	12.0	15.0	15.0	18.0	15.0	21.0	28.0
ANESTHESIOLOGY	10.0	14.0	15.0	20.0	20.0	20.0	30.0	31.5
CENSUS DIVISION								
NEW ENGLAND	20.0	20.0	24.0	30.0	25.0	30.0	40.0	47.0
MIDDLE ATLANTIC	20.0	23.2	28.0	30.0	30.0	30.0	50.0	47.0
EAST NORTH CENTRAL	27.0	29.6	30.0	34.0	35.0	40.0	50.0	60.0
WEST NORTH CENTRAL	30.0	30.0	33.0	35.0	35.0	46.0	76.0	64.0
SOUTH ATLANTIC	28.0	31.6	30.0	40.0	35.5	44.0	50.0	60.5
EAST SOUTH CENTRAL	33.0	31.0	40.0	45.0	40.0	44.0	58.0	70.5
WEST SOUTH CENTRAL	33.0	35.0	40.0	40.0	40.0	45.0	62.0	80.0
MOUNTAIN	30.5	30.0	35.0	40.0	40.0	44.0	49.0	63.0
PACIFIC	32.0	35.0	40.0	40.0	40.0	45.0	58.0	60.0
TYPE OF PRACTICE								
SOLO	25.0	28.0	30.0	35.0	38.0	40.0	50.0	59.0
NON-SOLO	30.0	30.0	33.0	40.0	31.5	40.0	60.0	64.0
LOCATION								
NONMETROPOLITAN	30.0	30.0	34.0	40.0	43.0	45.0	50.0	60.0
METROPOLITAN								
LESS THAN 1,000,000	30.0	30.0	32.0	40.0	40.0	40.0	56.0	62.0
1,000,000 AND OVER	24.0	28.0	30.0	33.5	30.0	38.0	54.0	57.0
PHYSICIAN AGE								
LESS THAN 36 YEARS	12.0	19.1	20.0	22.0	21.0	30.0	40.0	47.0
36-45 YEARS	30.0	31.0	35.0	40.0	40.0	45.0	53.5	63.0
46-55 YEARS	30.0	35.0	38.0	40.0	43.0	45.0	66.0	69.0
56-65 YEARS	25.0	28.0	33.0	35.0	40.0	40.0	53.0	63.0
66 OR MORE YEARS	17.0	18.0	19.0	20.0	25.0	28.0	45.0	46.0

SOURCE: 1981-82, AMA SOCIOECONOMIC MONITORING SYSTEM CORE SURVEYS; 1973-79, AMA PERIODIC SURVEYS OF PHYSICIANS.

*DATA, OTHER THAN IN THE SPECIALTY BREAKDOWN, ARE BASED ON RESPONSES FROM PHYSICIANS IN ALL SPECIALTIES. SEE APPENDIX FOR INFORMATION ON DEFINITIONS AND COMPUTATION PROCEDURES.

**CAUTION SHOULD BE OBSERVED IN COMPARING 1981 AND 1982 RESULTS WITH RESULTS FOR PREVIOUS YEARS BECAUSE OF CHANGES IN METHODOLOGY MADE IN THE TRANSITION FROM THE PERIODIC SURVEYS OF PHYSICIANS TO THE SOCIOECONOMIC MONITORING SYSTEM.

TABLE 37. MEANS OF SELECTED COMPONENTS OF PROFESSIONAL EXPENSES (IN THOUSANDS OF DOLLARS), 1982*

	NON-PHYSICIAN PAYROLL	OFFICE EXPENSES	MEDICAL SUPPLIES	PROFESSIONAL LIABILITY INSURANCE	MEDICAL EQUIPMENT
ALL PHYSICIANS	30.4	17.5	7.8	5.8	4.9
SPECIALTY					
GENERAL/FAMILY PRACTICE	31.5	17.7	11.2	3.5	4.3
INTERNAL MEDICINE	29.4	18.9	7.6	3.7	5.5
SURGERY	38.9	22.1	8.7	9.9	7.2
PEDIATRICS	25.8	17.6	7.8	2.9	2.6
OBSTETRICS/GYNECOLOGY	46.3	24.6	9.5	10.9	7.2
RADIOLOGY	24.7	12.6	8.5	4.9	6.7
PSYCHIATRY	11.4	13.3	1.6	1.7	1.7
ANESTHESIOLOGY	26.3	6.6	0.9	10.1	1.8
CENSUS DIVISION					
NEW ENGLAND	29.0	13.4	4.6	5.5	3.6
MIDDLE ATLANTIC	19.6	16.8	5.1	7.4	3.1
EAST NORTH CENTRAL	27.5	14.3	6.8	5.4	4.2
WEST NORTH CENTRAL	37.9	17.6	9.8	5.2	4.9
SOUTH ATLANTIC	32.4	18.3	7.5	5.7	4.9
EAST SOUTH CENTRAL	36.9	17.3	8.7	4.6	5.3
WEST SOUTH CENTRAL	39.3	22.8	12.1	4.2	7.3
MOUNTAIN	30.2	15.0	8.2	5.6	7.2
PACIFIC	28.4	19.5	7.8	6.7	5.1
TYPE OF PRACTICE					
SOLO	25.9	17.0	7.0	5.5	4.6
NON-SOLO	36.3	18.2	8.7	6.1	5.3
LOCATION					
NONMETROPOLITAN	31.6	17.2	7.9	5.6	5.0
METROPOLITAN					
LESS THAN 1,000,000	30.0	17.3	7.6	5.7	4.9
1,000,000 AND OVER	25.3	20.0	7.6	7.0	4.9
PHYSICIAN AGE					
LESS THAN 36 YEARS	18.9	13.3	6.0	4.4	3.7
36-45 YEARS	31.0	17.4	7.5	6.2	6.1
46-55 YEARS	35.5	20.4	9.4	6.3	5.3
56-65 YEARS	31.7	18.4	7.7	5.8	4.5
66 OR MORE YEARS	26.1	13.0	6.6	4.3	2.5

SOURCE: 1983 AMA SOCIOECONOMIC MONITORING SYSTEM CORE SURVEY.

*DATA EXCLUDE EMPLOYEE PHYSICIANS. DATA, OTHER THAN IN THE SPECIALTY BREAKDOWN, ARE BASED ON INFORMATION FROM PHYSICIANS IN ALL SPECIALTIES. SEE APPENDIX FOR INFORMATION ON DEFINITIONS AND COMPUTATION PROCEDURES.

TABLE 37 (CONTINUED). STANDARD ERRORS OF MEANS OF SELECTED COMPONENTS OF PROFESSIONAL EXPENSES (IN THOUSANDS OF DOLLARS), 1982*

	NON-PHYSICIAN PAYROLL	OFFICE EXPENSES	MEDICAL SUPPLIES	PROFESSIONAL LIABILITY INSURANCE	MEDICAL EQUIPMENT
ALL PHYSICIANS	0.87	0.51	0.31	0.14	0.26
SPECIALTY					
GENERAL/FAMILY PRACTICE	1.56	1.11	0.62	0.19	0.35
INTERNAL MEDICINE	1.61	1.08	0.59	0.26	0.88
SURGERY	2.30	1.16	0.66	0.35	0.69
PEDIATRICS	2.20	1.93	0.78	0.31	0.36
OBSTETRICS/GYNECOLOGY	3.53	2.84	1.13	0.58	1.28
RADIOLOGY	4.17	2.37	1.91	0.35	1.53
PSYCHIATRY	1.44	1.32	0.58	0.13	0.24
ANESTHESIOLOGY	4.63	1.32	0.44	0.59	0.42
CENSUS DIVISION					
NEW ENGLAND	4.07	1.51	0.64	0.56	0.65
MIDDLE ATLANTIC	1.41	1.56	0.69	0.45	0.41
EAST NORTH CENTRAL	1.63	0.92	0.64	0.30	0.43
WEST NORTH CENTRAL	4.20	1.90	1.53	0.50	0.79
SOUTH ATLANTIC	2.23	1.27	0.62	0.35	0.73
EAST SOUTH CENTRAL	3.57	1.91	1.17	0.39	0.67
WEST SOUTH CENTRAL	2.67	1.81	1.24	0.28	1.17
MOUNTAIN	3.36	1.46	1.32	0.49	1.49
PACIFIC	2.33	1.41	0.82	0.36	0.66
TYPE OF PRACTICE					
SOLO	0.86	0.60	0.37	0.18	0.32
NON-SOLO	1.65	0.88	0.51	0.21	0.44
LOCATION					
NONMETROPOLITAN	1.25	0.69	0.41	0.18	0.37
METROPOLITAN					
LESS THAN 1,000,000	1.18	0.86	0.51	0.23	0.40
1,000,000 AND OVER	3.40	1.56	1.07	0.51	1.00
PHYSICIAN AGE					
LESS THAN 36 YEARS	1.29	0.93	0.60	0.34	0.45
36-45 YEARS	1.65	0.93	0.50	0.24	0.55
46-55 YEARS	1.99	1.03	0.77	0.29	0.45
56-65 YEARS	1.71	1.23	0.65	0.29	0.67
66 OR MORE YEARS	2.38	1.47	0.79	0.37	0.33

SOURCE: 1983 AMA SOCIOECONOMIC MONITORING SYSTEM CORE SURVEY.

*DATA EXCLUDE EMPLOYEE PHYSICIANS. DATA, OTHER THAN IN THE SPECIALTY BREAKDOWN, ARE BASED ON INFORMATION FROM PHYSICIANS IN ALL SPECIALTIES. SEE APPENDIX FOR INFORMATION ON DEFINITIONS AND COMPUTATION PROCEDURES.

TABLE 38. MEAN NET INCOME FROM MEDICAL PRACTICE (IN THOUSANDS OF DOLLARS), 1982*

	ALL PHYSICIANS**	SPECIALTY								
		GP/FP	INT MED	SURG	PED	OB/GYN	RAD	PSYCH	ANES	PATH
ALL PHYSICIANS	99.5	71.9	86.8	130.5	70.3	115.8	136.8	76.5	131.4	114.4
CENSUS DIVISION										
NEW ENGLAND	82.2	60.9	70.8	99.3	63.1	123.5	93.9	71.0	126.9	.
MIDDLE ATLANTIC	91.1	60.3	86.0	133.5	58.2	101.5	103.7	76.1	110.2	80.2
EAST NORTH CENTRAL	106.2	76.5	88.8	143.9	68.5	112.1	152.6	87.6	142.4	122.9
WEST NORTH CENTRAL	106.5	75.3	93.5	147.4	80.8	113.8	155.5	81.3	144.7	.
SOUTH ATLANTIC	97.9	64.0	86.3	132.8	73.0	107.3	144.1	66.3	133.7	130.8
EAST SOUTH CENTRAL	106.8	83.2	93.7	116.4	75.4	124.5	178.9	.	136.0	.
WEST SOUTH CENTRAL	118.7	91.5	106.8	162.1	74.3	130.9	153.4	68.5	140.4	100.7
MOUNTAIN	95.8	73.2	62.8	108.7	.	143.8	112.3	109.1	130.1	.
PACIFIC	92.9	61.2	85.3	110.0	75.6	116.2	133.5	70.1	115.6	147.6
TYPE OF PRACTICE										
SOLO	93.4	68.5	86.3	120.4	75.9	113.1	124.5	77.7	123.7	117.3
NON-SOLO	104.0	76.1	87.3	140.9	68.1	118.4	138.2	74.5	134.6	114.0
LOCATION										
NONMETROPOLITAN	95.9	72.4	86.6	129.7	67.7	117.7	132.6	72.4	117.2	107.1
METROPOLITAN										
LESS THAN 1,000,000	105.8	69.2	88.4	135.2	73.5	115.9	142.2	80.9	144.7	118.5
1,000,000 AND OVER	95.9	79.8	83.9	114.7	70.8	106.8	135.1	81.3	124.1	.
EMPLOYMENT STATUS										
SELF-EMPLOYED	109.0	76.1	95.7	138.6	77.9	121.1	157.7	82.1	142.5	141.3
EMPLOYEE	71.5	51.7	64.3	80.8	57.0	80.7	93.6	62.0	97.4	78.5
PHYSICIAN AGE										
LESS THAN 36 YEARS	73.3	65.2	63.1	91.5	59.4	86.3	93.6	54.0	110.7	77.6
36-45 YEARS	108.2	75.2	95.2	145.2	68.4	120.5	144.3	72.1	127.6	113.5
46-55 YEARS	116.5	90.1	110.3	145.7	81.9	125.7	143.9	91.2	143.5	128.5
56-65 YEARS	99.5	71.7	83.4	122.7	74.9	121.7	153.4	76.6	141.6	121.8
66 OR MORE YEARS	64.3	51.9	64.1	76.4	.	57.5	103.1	64.9	.	.

SOURCE: 1983 AMA SOCIOECONOMIC MONITORING SYSTEM CORE SURVEY.

*SEE APPENDIX FOR INFORMATION ON DEFINITIONS AND COMPUTATION PROCEDURES.
**INCLUDES PHYSICIANS IN SPECIALTIES NOT LISTED SEPARATELY.
. INDICATES FEWER THAN TEN OBSERVATIONS.

TABLE 38 (CONTINUED). STANDARD ERROR OF MEAN NET INCOME FROM MEDICAL PRACTICE (IN THOUSANDS OF DOLLARS), 1982*

SPECIALTY

	ALL PHYSICIANS**	GP/FP	INT MED	SURG	PED	OB/GYN	RAD	PSYCH	ANES	PATH
ALL PHYSICIANS	1.23	1.88	2.38	3.85	2.69	4.69	4.39	2.82	4.53	6.96
CENSUS DIVISION										
NEW ENGLAND	3.42	8.11	5.77	9.73	6.72	12.97	14.39	11.18	10.29	.
MIDDLE ATLANTIC	3.11	5.09	6.34	11.60	4.93	13.03	8.51	7.24	8.08	8.84
EAST NORTH CENTRAL	3.16	5.42	5.56	11.00	6.03	10.02	10.13	7.21	10.20	19.41
WEST NORTH CENTRAL	4.88	5.74	9.73	14.01	14.42	24.63	18.01	9.13	16.70	.
SOUTH ATLANTIC	2.78	3.72	5.60	7.70	6.25	11.06	9.01	5.10	16.68	14.59
EAST SOUTH CENTRAL	4.33	6.31	9.86	9.75	4.87	16.18	20.22	.	11.44	.
WEST SOUTH CENTRAL	5.28	6.54	8.39	16.76	14.08	14.75	21.23	7.74	12.59	22.44
MOUNTAIN	4.87	6.93	10.19	13.99	.	24.31	15.48	18.41	16.65	.
PACIFIC	2.70	3.56	6.23	7.19	6.46	11.08	9.84	4.59	16.15	22.13
TYPE OF PRACTICE										
SOLO	1.91	2.56	3.85	5.23	6.26	7.31	11.40	3.18	8.75	18.93
NON-SOLO	1.60	2.74	3.01	5.60	2.84	5.94	4.72	5.23	5.28	7.50
LOCATION										
NONMETROPOLITAN	1.72	2.46	3.61	5.81	3.67	6.56	6.05	3.22	6.74	7.99
METROPOLITAN										
LESS THAN 1,000,000	2.04	2.95	3.57	5.63	4.45	8.35	7.32	5.35	6.28	11.40
1,000,000 AND OVER	3.41	8.25	6.11	11.12	8.33	9.00	12.74	9.59	15.92	.
EMPLOYMENT STATUS										
SELF-EMPLOYED	1.52	2.10	2.93	4.29	3.76	5.18	5.34	3.72	5.29	10.11
EMPLOYEE	1.40	3.41	3.28	5.21	2.88	7.16	4.58	2.53	6.14	5.42
PHYSICIAN AGE										
LESS THAN 36 YEARS	2.09	3.10	3.53	9.01	4.82	14.20	10.67	3.62	8.86	18.21
36-45 YEARS	2.39	3.38	4.53	7.36	4.52	7.69	6.88	3.75	7.57	10.02
46-55 YEARS	2.54	4.37	5.14	7.25	6.83	10.81	7.17	6.01	8.89	12.25
56-65 YEARS	2.63	4.21	5.25	7.09	4.97	7.22	12.92	7.40	10.58	19.66
66 OR MORE YEARS	3.28	4.47	8.38	9.00	.	13.48	23.24	8.08	.	.

SOURCE: 1983 AMA SOCIOECONOMIC MONITORING SYSTEM CORE SURVEY.

*SEE APPENDIX FOR INFORMATION ON DEFINITIONS AND COMPUTATION PROCEDURES.
**INCLUDES PHYSICIANS IN SPECIALTIES NOT LISTED SEPARATELY.
. INDICATES FEWER THAN TEN OBSERVATIONS.

TABLE 39. MEAN NET INCOME FROM MEDICAL PRACTICE (IN THOUSANDS OF DOLLARS), 1973-75, 1977-79, 1981-82*

	1973	1974	1975	1977	1978	1979	1981**	1982**
ALL PHYSICIANS	48.6	52.0	56.4	61.2	65.5	78.4	93.0	99.5
SPECIALTY								
GENERAL/FAMILY PRACTICE	41.9	44.7	45.4	51.1	54.6	62.0	72.2	71.9
INTERNAL MEDICINE	47.8	51.4	57.0	61.5	63.8	76.2	85.1	86.8
SURGERY	57.4	60.5	68.2	74.0	82.6	96.0	118.6	130.5
PEDIATRICS	41.1	42.1	44.3	48.2	51.2	60.4	65.1	70.3
OBSTETRICS/GYNECOLOGY	55.4	61.7	63.3	69.9	70.3	91.8	110.8	115.8
RADIOLOGY	59.5	63.8	75.2	76.7	81.5	98.0	116.9	136.8
PSYCHIATRY	38.4	41.3	44.8	48.2	50.2	62.6	70.6	76.5
ANESTHESIOLOGY	48.1	54.4	57.1	65.5	74.2	91.4	118.6	131.4
CENSUS DIVISION								
NEW ENGLAND	44.2	46.3	47.2	53.1	54.9	66.6	85.0	82.2
MIDDLE ATLANTIC	43.8	47.7	53.2	55.9	59.1	73.2	85.6	91.1
EAST NORTH CENTRAL	50.5	54.2	59.9	62.7	69.9	81.2	100.9	106.2
WEST NORTH CENTRAL	51.5	53.6	56.6	61.1	70.2	79.4	87.4	106.5
SOUTH ATLANTIC	50.3	54.4	58.2	61.8	64.9	79.8	92.6	97.9
EAST SOUTH CENTRAL	53.3	58.4	65.5	68.2	79.7	87.0	97.4	106.8
WEST SOUTH CENTRAL	52.8	57.7	61.4	67.9	70.9	85.8	101.6	118.7
MOUNTAIN	47.4	49.5	54.7	57.5	61.8	73.5	92.6	95.8
PACIFIC	48.1	50.9	54.8	63.6	64.9	78.6	91.7	92.9
TYPE OF PRACTICE								
SOLO	45.3	48.5	51.6	56.3	61.3	75.8	88.4	93.4
NON-SOLO	52.8	55.6	61.1	68.3	69.9	80.7	96.6	104.0
LOCATION								
NONMETROPOLITAN	46.9	48.5	50.2	56.7	64.8	74.1	89.7	95.9
METROPOLITAN								
LESS THAN 1,000,000	50.3	53.7	58.8	63.2	67.4	78.8	99.6	105.8
1,000,000 AND OVER	47.5	51.5	55.6	60.6	63.9	78.8	87.6	95.9
PHYSICIAN AGE								
LESS THAN 36 YEARS	32.8	40.6	43.7	49.6	49.0	64.3	62.5	73.3
36-45 YEARS	51.9	57.1	62.9	69.9	70.1	87.5	98.1	108.2
46-55 YEARS	55.0	58.9	62.3	67.7	76.2	87.1	110.8	116.5
56-65 YEARS	48.3	49.3	54.1	58.7	65.3	75.9	95.6	99.5
66 OR MORE YEARS	31.9	34.0	35.0	36.8	44.4	54.9	68.3	64.3

SOURCE: 1981-82, AMA SOCIOECONOMIC MONITORING SYSTEM CORE SURVEYS; 1973-79, AMA PERIODIC SURVEYS OF PHYSICIANS.

*DATA, OTHER THAN IN THE SPECIALTY BREAKDOWN, ARE BASED ON RESPONSES FROM PHYSICIANS IN ALL SPECIALTIES. SEE APPENDIX FOR INFORMATION ON DEFINITIONS AND COMPUTATION PROCEDURES.

**CAUTION SHOULD BE OBSERVED IN COMPARING 1981 AND 1982 RESULTS WITH RESULTS FOR PREVIOUS YEARS BECAUSE OF CHANGES IN METHODOLOGY MADE IN THE TRANSITION FROM THE PERIODIC SURVEYS OF PHYSICIANS TO THE SOCIOECONOMIC MONITORING SYSTEM.

TABLE 39 (CONTINUED). STANDARD ERROR OF MEAN NET INCOME FROM MEDICAL PRACTICE (IN THOUSANDS OF DOLLARS). 1973-75, 1977-79, 1981-82*

	1973	1974	1975	1977	1978	1979	1981**	1982**
ALL PHYSICIANS	0.40	0.43	0.48	0.57	0.65	0.71	1.53	1.23
SPECIALTY								
GENERAL/FAMILY PRACTICE	0.70	0.82	0.75	1.05	1.11	1.30	3.34	1.88
INTERNAL MEDICINE	0.95	0.97	1.12	1.30	1.38	1.57	3.28	2.38
SURGERY	1.01	1.00	1.24	1.42	1.82	1.67	4.04	3.85
PEDIATRICS	1.22	1.15	1.57	1.52	1.61	1.54	4.86	2.69
OBSTETRICS/GYNECOLOGY	1.64	1.78	1.73	2.14	2.16	2.87	9.16	4.69
RADIOLOGY	1.72	2.17	2.40	2.88	2.90	5.39	4.05	4.39
PSYCHIATRY	0.90	1.09	1.01	1.28	1.37	2.01	2.54	2.82
ANESTHESIOLOGY	1.39	1.29	1.65	2.78	2.71	2.62	4.97	4.53
CENSUS DIVISION								
NEW ENGLAND	1.37	1.51	1.61	1.84	2.08	2.11	7.51	3.42
MIDDLE ATLANTIC	0.86	0.91	1.17	1.23	1.64	1.83	4.46	3.11
EAST NORTH CENTRAL	1.04	1.08	1.26	1.39	1.74	1.70	4.58	3.16
WEST NORTH CENTRAL	1.69	1.76	1.68	2.00	2.58	2.12	3.74	4.88
SOUTH ATLANTIC	1.01	1.18	1.18	1.48	1.64	1.67	3.19	2.78
EAST SOUTH CENTRAL	1.92	2.19	2.46	2.71	3.41	4.01	5.56	4.33
WEST SOUTH CENTRAL	1.36	1.63	2.00	2.33	2.26	2.75	4.11	5.28
MOUNTAIN	1.65	1.60	1.93	2.31	2.23	2.47	4.74	4.87
PACIFIC	0.98	1.03	1.00	1.40	1.30	1.70	3.47	2.70
TYPE OF PRACTICE								
SOLO	0.54	0.61	0.67	0.72	0.92	1.07	2.41	1.91
NON-SOLO	0.59	0.60	0.68	0.90	0.90	0.95	1.95	1.60
LOCATION								
NONMETROPOLITAN	1.14	1.14	1.26	1.68	1.70	2.36	1.95	1.72
METROPOLITAN								
LESS THAN 1,000,000	0.64	0.67	0.76	0.91	1.07	1.05	2.84	2.04
1,000,000 AND OVER	0.58	0.64	0.70	0.82	0.91	1.05	4.23	3.41
PHYSICIAN AGE								
LESS THAN 36 YEARS	1.33	1.16	1.44	1.30	1.64	1.59	2.20	2.09
36-45 YEARS	0.68	0.77	0.87	1.09	1.22	1.37	2.49	2.39
46-55 YEARS	0.72	0.80	0.91	1.01	1.29	1.47	3.59	2.54
56-65 YEARS	0.90	0.84	0.93	1.33	1.32	1.47	4.06	2.63
66 OR MORE YEARS	0.94	1.18	1.13	1.38	1.33	1.71	3.02	3.28

SOURCE: 1981-82, AMA SOCIOECONOMIC MONITORING SYSTEM CORE SURVEYS; 1973-79, AMA PERIODIC SURVEYS OF PHYSICIANS.

*DATA, OTHER THAN IN THE SPECIALTY BREAKDOWN, ARE BASED ON RESPONSES FROM PHYSICIANS IN ALL SPECIALTIES. SEE APPENDIX FOR INFORMATION ON DEFINITIONS AND COMPUTATION PROCEDURES.
**CAUTION SHOULD BE OBSERVED IN COMPARING 1981 AND 1982 RESULTS WITH RESULTS FOR PREVIOUS YEARS BECAUSE OF CHANGES IN METHODOLOGY MADE IN THE TRANSITION FROM THE PERIODIC SURVEYS OF PHYSICIANS TO THE SOCIOECONOMIC MONITORING SYSTEM.

TABLE 40. MEDIAN NET INCOME FROM MEDICAL PRACTICE (IN THOUSANDS OF DOLLARS), 1982*

SPECIALTY

	ALL PHYSICIANS**	GP/FP	INT MED	SURG	PED	OB/GYN	RAD	PSYCH	ANES	PATH
ALL PHYSICIANS	85.0	63.0	75.0	112.0	63.0	110.0	127.5	69.0	120.0	98.5
CENSUS DIVISION										
NEW ENGLAND	72.0	50.0	63.0	91.0	53.5	130.0	90.0	60.0	125.0	.
MIDDLE ATLANTIC	75.0	53.0	74.0	118.0	54.5	92.5	105.0	68.0	113.5	75.0
EAST NORTH CENTRAL	92.0	70.5	80.0	120.0	58.0	114.5	154.5	77.0	126.0	102.5
WEST NORTH CENTRAL	91.0	62.0	98.0	124.0	62.0	105.5	164.0	70.0	130.0	.
SOUTH ATLANTIC	81.5	58.0	75.0	119.0	74.0	105.0	140.0	59.5	139.0	111.0
EAST SOUTH CENTRAL	95.0	73.5	82.0	114.5	74.0	117.0	189.5	.	131.0	.
WEST SOUTH CENTRAL	100.0	83.0	98.0	136.0	58.0	117.5	145.0	65.0	130.0	84.5
MOUNTAIN	83.0	70.0	48.0	85.0	.	144.0	107.5	95.0	130.0	.
PACIFIC	80.0	59.0	74.0	100.0	70.0	113.0	120.0	70.0	101.5	129.0
TYPE OF PRACTICE										
SOLO	79.0	60.0	72.0	100.0	73.0	105.5	120.0	73.0	114.5	125.0
NON-SOLO	90.0	66.0	78.0	120.0	60.0	111.5	128.0	65.0	126.0	98.0
LOCATION										
NONMETROPOLITAN	81.0	63.0	73.0	107.0	63.0	110.0	120.5	64.5	105.0	91.0
METROPOLITAN										
LESS THAN 1,000,000	90.0	63.0	80.0	120.0	65.5	110.0	138.0	74.0	139.5	102.5
1,000,000 AND OVER	80.0	77.5	73.0	99.0	55.0	109.0	117.0	70.0	110.5	.
EMPLOYMENT STATUS										
SELF-EMPLOYED	95.0	70.0	86.5	120.0	73.0	113.5	153.0	76.0	133.5	130.0
EMPLOYEE	65.0	47.5	58.5	74.0	55.0	77.0	88.0	60.0	92.0	76.5
PHYSICIAN AGE										
LESS THAN 36 YEARS	62.0	60.0	55.0	75.0	52.0	70.0	75.0	54.0	103.0	64.0
36-45 YEARS	94.0	70.0	76.5	120.0	62.5	115.0	140.0	68.0	130.0	99.0
46-55 YEARS	100.0	81.0	102.0	130.0	79.0	108.5	131.0	80.0	130.0	128.0
56-65 YEARS	85.5	60.0	80.0	101.5	73.5	122.5	160.0	64.0	130.0	100.0
66 OR MORE YEARS	54.0	42.5	61.0	66.5	.	68.0	99.5	53.5	.	.

SOURCE: 1983 AMA SOCIOECONOMIC MONITORING SYSTEM CORE SURVEY.

*SEE APPENDIX FOR INFORMATION ON DEFINITIONS AND COMPUTATION PROCEDURES.
**INCLUDES PHYSICIANS IN SPECIALTIES NOT LISTED SEPARATELY.
. INDICATES FEWER THAN TEN OBSERVATIONS.

TABLE 41. MEDIAN NET INCOME FROM MEDICAL PRACTICE (IN THOUSANDS OF DOLLARS), 1973-75, 1977-79, 1981-82*

	1973	1974	1975	1977	1978	1979	1981**	1982**
ALL PHYSICIANS	45.0	50.0	50.0	56.0	60.0	70.0	78.0	85.0
SPECIALTY								
GENERAL/FAMILY PRACTICE	40.0	40.5	42.0	48.0	50.0	58.0	60.0	63.0
INTERNAL MEDICINE	45.0	50.0	52.0	59.0	60.0	70.0	74.5	75.0
SURGERY	54.0	56.0	60.0	70.0	75.0	86.0	100.0	112.0
PEDIATRICS	40.0	40.0	42.0	48.0	50.0	58.0	57.0	63.0
OBSTETRICS/GYNECOLOGY	52.0	58.5	60.0	65.0	69.5	82.0	96.0	110.0
RADIOLOGY	60.0	60.0	71.0	72.0	79.5	86.0	110.0	127.5
PSYCHIATRY	37.0	40.0	43.0	46.0	50.0	60.0	63.0	69.0
ANESTHESIOLOGY	50.0	52.0	54.5	64.0	72.0	84.5	110.0	120.0
CENSUS DIVISION								
NEW ENGLAND	40.0	43.0	44.0	50.0	50.0	60.0	67.5	72.0
MIDDLE ATLANTIC	40.0	45.0	48.0	53.0	52.0	62.0	70.0	75.0
EAST NORTH CENTRAL	47.0	50.0	54.0	60.0	63.0	75.0	84.5	92.0
WEST NORTH CENTRAL	47.0	50.0	50.0	56.0	64.0	72.0	80.0	91.0
SOUTH ATLANTIC	48.0	50.0	53.0	56.0	60.0	73.0	78.0	81.5
EAST SOUTH CENTRAL	50.0	55.0	60.0	67.0	75.0	80.0	84.0	95.0
WEST SOUTH CENTRAL	50.0	52.0	57.0	61.0	66.0	75.0	87.5	100.0
MOUNTAIN	45.5	48.5	50.0	54.0	58.0	70.0	80.0	83.0
PACIFIC	44.0	48.0	50.0	60.0	60.0	70.0	80.0	80.0
TYPE OF PRACTICE								
SOLO	41.0	45.0	46.0	50.0	55.0	66.0	72.0	79.0
NON-SOLO	50.0	52.0	57.0	62.0	65.0	75.0	81.0	90.0
LOCATION								
NONMETROPOLITAN	45.0	45.0	45.0	50.5	60.0	65.0	76.0	81.0
METROPOLITAN								
LESS THAN 1,000,000	47.0	50.0	53.0	60.0	60.0	72.0	80.0	90.0
1,000,000 AND OVER	44.0	49.0	50.0	55.0	60.0	70.0	75.0	80.0
PHYSICIAN AGE								
LESS THAN 36 YEARS	29.0	37.0	40.0	45.0	45.0	57.0	54.0	62.0
36-45 YEARS	49.0	53.0	60.0	64.0	63.0	80.0	81.0	94.0
46-55 YEARS	50.0	54.0	59.0	62.0	70.0	80.0	95.0	100.0
56-65 YEARS	45.0	47.0	50.0	52.0	60.0	69.0	80.0	85.5
66 OR MORE YEARS	28.0	30.0	30.0	34.0	40.0	50.0	60.0	54.0

SOURCE: 1981-82, AMA SOCIOECONOMIC MONITORING SYSTEM CORE SURVEYS; 1973-79, AMA PERIODIC SURVEYS OF PHYSICIANS.

*DATA, OTHER THAN IN THE SPECIALTY BREAKDOWN, ARE BASED ON RESPONSES FROM PHYSICIANS IN ALL SPECIALTIES. SEE APPENDIX FOR INFORMATION ON DEFINITIONS AND COMPUTATION PROCEDURES.

**CAUTION SHOULD BE OBSERVED IN COMPARING 1981 AND 1982 RESULTS FOR PREVIOUS YEARS BECAUSE OF CHANGES IN METHODOLOGY MADE IN THE TRANSITION FROM THE PERIODIC SURVEYS OF PHYSICIANS TO THE SOCIOECONOMIC MONITORING SYSTEM.

Appendix A

SMS QUESTIONNAIRE SUMMARY

This summary includes questions contained in the screener and main questionnaire portions of SMS surveys conducted in 1982. These questions were identical in each of the four surveys during the year. In the main questionnaire, only questions applicable to the physician's specialty and type of practice are asked of any individual physician. In addition, the summary includes selected questions from core survey expansions of the main questionnaire and selected special topics questions on which SMS Reports in 1982 and 1983 and information in Socio-economic Characteristics of Medical Practice 1983 have been based.

Following is a listing of subjects covered in the main questionnaire, the core survey main questionnaire expansion and special topics portions of SMS surveys included in the summary.

MAIN QUESTIONNAIRE

- Practice Activities: Hours and Services Per Week
- Selected Procedures: Number Delivered and Fees
- Hospital Utilization
- Quarterly Income and Expenses

CORE AND SPECIAL TOPICS QUESTIONS

- Physician Financial Arrangements with Hospitals
- Ambulatory Surgery
- Medical Technology Diffusion
- 1982 Core Survey Questions: 1981 Income and Expenses and Waiting Time
- Non-Physician Personnel
- Malpractice Claims Experience
- Physician/Hospital Relations
- Impact of the Economy on Physicians
- Physician Responses to Competition
- 1983 Core Survey Questions: Type of Practice, 1982 Income and Expenses and Waiting Time

Since the entire questionnaire is quite lengthy, some questions are paraphrased in the summary. Parts of questions that are paraphrased are indicated with square brackets. Questions that have been dropped from the main questionnaire during 1982 and for which information has never been reported are omitted from the summary.

1. Is [MASTERFILE SPECIALTY] your primary specialty, that is, the specialty from which you derive most of your medical income?*

    [IF "YES", GO TO Q. 2]
    a. What is your primary medical specialty?

2. During a typical week, do you provide patient care for 20 hours a week or more? Patient care includes seeing patients, performing surgery, as well as related patient services performed by anesthesiologists, radiologists and pathologists.

3. Are you currently a full-time, salaried employee of a federal agency such as the U.S. Public Health Service, Veteran's Administration or a military service?

MAIN QUESTIONAIRE

PRACTICE ACTIVITIES: HOURS AND SERVICES PER WEEK

All specialties except psychiatry, radiology, anesthesiology and pathology

4. During [your last complete week of practice], how many hours did you spend. . .
    a. In the office seeing patients? Please include time spent in all offices if practice includes multiple offices.
    b. In the operating, labor or delivery room? Please include waiting time before surgery.
    c. Making hospital rounds, including visits to newborn infants?
    d. In the hospital emergency room?
    e. In outpatient clinics?
    f. On house calls and with patients in nursing homes, convalescent homes or other extended care facilities?
    g. Having telephone conversations with patients or their families, consulting with other physicians and providing other services to patient such as interpreting lab tests and X-rays? Do not include time reported in other activities.
    h. In administrative activities connected with your practice and other medical facilities, as well as any other professional activities that did not involve patient care? These activities include medical staff functions, supervising residents and interns, teaching, lecturing, professional reading, writing and research.

5. Altogether, during that week, that amounts to [TOTAL HOURS] spent working at medical and administrative activities. Is that correct?**

---

 * MASTERFILE SPECIALTY is from information obtained from the AMA Physician Masterfile while selecting the sample.
** TOTAL HOURS is computed as the sum of responses to individual parts of Question 4 If the physician answers "no" to Question 5, then Question 4 is repeated.

6. During [your last complete week of practice], how many. . .
   a. Patients did you personally see in the office, including out-patient surgery performed in the office?
      1. How many of these patients were new patients?
   b. Operations, deliveries and assists did you perform in the hospital?
   c. In-patient visits did you make on hospital rounds? Please count as one visit every time you saw a patient.
   d. Patients did you see in the emergency room?
   e. Patients did you see in outpatient clinics?
   f. Patients did you see on house calls or in nursing homes, convalescent homes or extended care facilities?

Psychiatry

7. During [your last complete week of practice], how many hours did you spend. . .
   a. In the office seeing patients? Please include time spent in all offices if practice includes multiple offices.
   b. In all other settings seeing individual patients?
   c. Seeing family or non-family groups? Include time spent in all settings as well as house calls?
   d. Supervising psychiatric treatment teams, consulting with other physicians and providing other services to patients, such as interpreting lab tests and X-rays? Do not include time reported in other activities.
   e. In administrative activities connected with your practice and other medical facilities, as well as any other professional activities that did not involve patient care? These activities include medical staff functions, supervising residents and interns, teaching, lecturing, professional reading, writing and research.

8. Altogether, during that week, that amounts to [TOTAL HOURS] spent working at medical and administrative activities. Is that correct?*

9. During [your last complete week of practice], how many hours did you spend. . .
   a. Sessions did you have with individual patients in the office?
   b. Sessions did you have with individual patients in all other settings?
   c. Sessions did you have with non-family groups?
   d. Sessions did you have with family groups?

Radiology

10. During [your last complete week of practice], how many hours did you spend. . .
    a. Reading films, including time spent preparing reports on films read?

---

* TOTAL HOURS is computed as the sum of responses to individual parts of Question 7. If the physician answers "no" to Question 8, then Question 7 is repeated.

b. Personally performing radiodiagnostic procedures?
c. Personally providing radiotherapy to patients?
d. Supervising technicians and other paraprofessionals?
e. In consultation with other physicians?
f. In administrative activities connected with your practice and other medical facilities, as well as any other professional activities that did not involve patient care? These activities include medical staff functions, supervising residents and interns, teaching, lecturing, professional reading, writing and research.

11. Altogether, during that week, that amounts to [TOTAL HOURS] spent working at medical and administrative activities. Is that correct?*

12. During [your last complete week of practice], how many. . .
a. Films did you read?
b. Radiodiagnostic procedures did you personally perform?
c. Patients did you personally provide with radiotherapy?
d. Radiological procedures were performed by technicians and paraprofessionals working under your supervision?
e. Consultations did you have with other physicians?

Anesthesiology

13. During [your last complete week of practice], how many hours did you spend. . .
a. Personally anesthetizing patients? Include waiting time before surgery.
b. Supervising nurse anesthetists?
c. Making pre-anesthesia visits, including histories and examinations?
d. Managing patients in intensive care units?
e. Seeing patients on hospital rounds? Do not include time spent making pre-anesthesia visits or managing patients in intensive care units.
f. Consulting with other physicians about their patients and providing any other services to patients, such as interpreting lab tests and X-rays?
g. In administrative activities connected with your practice and other medical facilities, as well as any other professional activities that did not involve patient care? These activities include medical staff functions, supervising residents and interns, teaching, lecturing, professional reading, writing and research.

14. Altogether, during that week, that amounts to [TOTAL HOURS] spent working at medical and administrative activities. Is that correct?**

---

* TOTAL HOURS is computed as the sum of responses to individual parts of Question 10. If the physician answers "no" to Question 11, then Question 10 is repeated.
** TOTAL HOURS is computed as the sum of responses to individual parts of Question 13. If the physician answers "no" to Question 14, then Question 13 is repeated.

15. During your last complete week of practice, how many...
    a. Patients did you personally anesthetize?
    b. Patients were anesthetized by nurse anesthetists under your supervision?
    c. Pre-anesthesia visits did you make?
    d. Patients did you manage in an intensive care unit?
    e. In-patient visits did you make on hospital rounds, not including pre-anesthesia visist to patients in intensive care units?

Pathology

16. During [your last complete week of practice], how many hours did you spend. . .
    a. In consultations during surgery, including time spent interpreting frozen sections?
    b. Examining surgical specimens other than consultations during surgery?
    c. Doing autopsies, including time to complete the study and write the report?
    d. Personally performing non-surgical laboratory procedures, including time to write any reports?
    e. Supervising technicians and paraprofessionals?
    f. In administrative activities connected with your practice and other medical facilities, as well as any other professional activities that did not involve patient care? These activities include medical staff functions, supervising residents and interns, teaching, lecturing, professional reading, writing and research.

17. Altogether, during that week, that amounts to [TOTAL HOURS] spent working at medical and administrative activities. Is that correct?*

18. During [your last complete week of practice], how many. . .
    a. Consultations during surgery did you perform?
    b. Surgical specimens did you examine other than frozen sections examined during surgical consultations?
    c. Autopsies did you perform?
    d. Non-surgical laboratory procedures did you personally perform?

SELECTED PROCEDURES: NUMBER DELIVERED AND FEES

All specialties except ophthalmology, psychiatry, radiology, anesthesiology and pathology

19. Does your practice provide at least some care on a fee-for-service basis?   [IF "NO", GO TO HOSPITAL UTILIZATION QUESTIONS]

20. What is your current usual fee for. . .
    a. An office visit with a new patient including an evaluation history, examination and/or treatment?

---

* TOTAL HOURS is computed as the sum of responses to individual parts of Question 16. If the physician answers "no" to Question 17, then Question 16 is repeated.

b. An office visit with an established patient including an examination and/or treatment of the same or new illness?

c. A follow-up medical visit in the hospital, when you charge a separate fee for hospital visits? This visit includes an examination, evaluation and/or treatment with a new or established patient, same illness.

21. During your most recent week of practice, about what percentage of your inpatient visits were included in the fee for surgical or obstetrical procedures?

Ophthalmology

22. What is your current usual fee for. . .
a. An office visit with a new patient to initiate an ophthalmological diagnostic and treatment program?

b. An office visit with an established patient to initate or continue an ophthalmological diagnostic and treatment program?

c. A follow-up medical visit in the hospital, when you charge a separate fee for hospital visits? This visit includes an examination, evaluation and/or treatment with a new or established patient, same illness.

23. During your most recent complete week of practice, about what percentage of your inpatient visits were included in the fee for surgical prcedures?

24. During the last month, did you perform an operation to remove a cataract?*
a. How many of these procedures did you perform in the last month?
b. What is your current usual fee for that procedure?

25. During the last month, did you prescribe and fit contact lenses, including medical supervision by adaptation?*
a. How many of these procedures did you perform in the last month?
b. What is your usual current fee for that procedure?

All specialties except pediatrics, ophthalmology, psychiatry, radiology, anesthesiology and pathology

26. During the last month, did you perform a periodic or annual type of exam with an adult established patient?*
a. How many of these exams did you perform during that month?
b. What is your current usual fee for that exam, excluding any lab or x-ray charges?

Pediatrics

27. During the last month, did you perform a periodic or annual type of exam with an established patient in early childhood?*
a. How many of these exams did you perform during that month?

---

*Parts a and b of the question are asked only if the response is "yes".

b. What is your current usual fee for that exam, excluding any lab or x-ray charges?

28. During the last month, did you provide routine newborn care in the hospital, including physician examination of the baby and discussions with the mother during the hospital stay?*
    a. How many of these examinations did you perform during that month?
    b. What is your current usual fee for the examination, excluding any lab or x-ray charges?

General/Family Practice and General Surgery

29. During the last month, did you perform an appendectomy?*
    a. How many appendectomies did you perform?
    b. What is your current usual fee for that procedure?

General/Family Practice and Obstetrics/Gynecology

30. During the last month, did you perform any vaginal deliveries which included antepartum and postpartum care?*
    a. How many of these deliveries did you perform during the last month?
    b. What is your current usual fee for complete obstetrical care leading to a vaginal delivery including antepartum care, vaginal delivery and postpartum care?

31. During the last month, did you perform any cesarean sections which included antepartum and postpartum care?*
    a. How many cesarean sections did you perform during the last month?
    b. What is your current usual fee for cesarean section with antepartum and postpartum care?

General/Family Practice and Internal Medicine

32. During the last month, how many electrocardiograms did you personally interpret?**
    a. What is the usual charge, including the fee for the use of the electrocardiograph, for an electrocardiogram including interpretation and report?

General Surgery and Obstetrics/Gynecology

33. During the last month, did you perform a total hysterectomy?*
    a. How many of these procedures did you perform during that month?
    b. What is your current usual fee for that procedure?

34. During the last month, did you perform a diagnostic dilation and curettage of the uterus?*

---

*Parts a and b of the question are asked only if the response is "yes".
**Part a of the question is not asked if the response is "none".

a. How many of these procedures did you perform during that month?
b. What is your current usual fee for that procedure?

General Surgery

35. During the last month, did you perform a single inguinal hernia
    repair on a person age 5 or older?*
    a. How many of these procedures did you perform during that month?
    b. What is your current usual fee for that procedure?

36. During the last month, did you perform a cholecystectomy?*
    a. How many of these procedures did you perform during that month?
    b. What is your current usual fee for that procedure?

Otalaryngology

37. During the last month, did you perform a tonsillectomy with an
    adenoidectomy on a child 12 years of age or under?*
    a. How many of these procedures did you perform during that month?
    b. What is your current usual fee for that procedure?

38. During the last month, did you perform a submucous resection of a
    nasal septum?*
    a. How many of these procedures did you perform during that month?
    b. What is your current usual fee for that procedure?

39. During the last month, did you perform a myringotomy?*
    a. How many of these procedures did you perform during that month?
    b. What is your current usual fee for that procedure?

40. During the last month, did you perform a rhinoplasty?*
    a. How many of these procedures did you perform during that month?
    b. What is your current usual fee for that procedure?

Orthopedic Surgery

41. During the last month, did you suture and perform a secondary
    repair of a torn, ruptured, or severed knee, collateral and
    cruciate ligaments?*
    a. How many of these procedures did you perform during that month?
    b. What is your current usual fee for that procedure?

42. During the last month, did you perform a total hip replacement?*
    a. How many of these procedures did you perform during that month?
    b. What is your current usual fee for that procedure?

43. During the last month, did you perform a laminectomy?*
    a. How many of these procedures did you perform during that month?
    b. What is your current usual fee for that procedure?

44. During the last month, did you treat a closed ulnar shaft fracture
    without manipulation?*

---

*Part a and b of the question are asked only if the response is "yes".

a. How many of these procedures did you perform during that month?
b. What is your current usual fee for that procedure?

Urology

45. During the last month, did you perform a transurethral resection of the prostate?*
    a. How many of these procedures did you perform during that month?
    b. What is your current usual fee for that procedure?

46. During the last month, did you perform a cystourethroscopy with urethral catheterization?*
    a. How many of these procedures did you perform during that month?
    b. What is your current usual fee for that procedure?

Psychiatry

47. What is your current usual fee for individual psychotherapy?
    a. How many minutes are there in a typical session?

48. What is your current usual fee per person for psychotherapy to a non-family group?
    a. How many minutes are there in a typical session?
    b. How many persons are there in a typical session?

49. What is your current usual fee for family psychotherapy?
    a. How many minutes are there in a typical session?

50. During the last month, did you perform a psychiatric diagnostic evaluation?**
    a. How many of these examinations did you perform during the last month?
    b. What is the current usual fee for that examination?

Radiology

51. During the last month, did you interpret or perform a radiologic exam of the upper gastrointestinal tract without K.U.B.?**
    a. Approximately how many of these procedures did you interpret or perform during the last month?
    b. What is the current usual charge for that procedure?
    c. Does that charge include laboratory and X-ray fees?

52. During the last month, did you interpret or perform a radiologic exam of the chest?**
    a. Approximately how many of these procedures did you interpret or perform during the last month?
    b. What is the current usual charge for that procedure?
    c. Does that charge include laboratory and X-ray fees?

---

*Part a and b of the question are asked only if the response is "yes".
**Parts a-c of this question are asked only if the response is "yes".

53. During the last month, did you interpret or perform a B-scan echography of the gall bladder?*
    a. Approximately how many of these procedures did you interpret or perform during the last month?
    b. What is the current usual charge for tha procedure?
    c. Does that charge include laboratory and X-ray fees?

54. During the last month, did you interpret or perform a computerized tomography of the head with intravenous contrast?*
    a. Approximately how many of these procedures did you interpret or perform during the last month?
    b. What is the current usual charge for that procedure?
    c. Does that charge include laboratory and X-ray fees?

55. During the last month, did you interpret or perform a complete abdominal series?*
    a. Approximately how many of these procedures did you interpret or perform during the last month?
    b. What is the current usual charge for that procedure?
    c. Does that charge include laboratory and X-ray fees?

56. During the last month, did you interpret or perform a bilateral mammograpy?*
    a. Approximately how many of these procedures did you interpret or perform during the last month?
    b. What is the current usual charge for that procedure?
    c. Does that charge include laboratory and X-ray fees?

Anesthesiology

57. Is your fee [for administering anesthesia] based upon both the complexity of the procedure and the number of units of anesthesia time required?**
    a. What is your current usual charge per unit of anesthesia time?
    b. How many minutes are there in a unit of anesthesia time?
    c. How much total anesthesia time did you bill for during your last complete week of practice?

58. During the last month, did you administer anesthesia for an inguinal hernia repair?***
    a. How many of these operationds did you administer anesthesia for during the last month?
    b. How many units are included in the base charge for that procedure, assuming no unusual complications and excluding the charge for anesthesia time?

59. During the last month, did you administer anesthesia for a total hysterectomy?***

---

*Parts a-c of this question are asked only if the response is "yes".
**Parts of this question and questions 58-62 are not asked if the response is "no".
***Parts a and b of the question are not asked if the response is "no".

a. How many of these operations did you administer anesthesia for during the last month?

b. How many units are included in the base charge for that procedure, assuming no unusual complications and <u>excluding</u> the charge for anesthesia time?

60. During the last month, did you administer anesthesia for a thoracotomy with lung resection?*

    a. How many of these operations did you administer anesthesia for during the last month?

    b. How many units are included in the base charge for that procedure, assuming no unusual complications and <u>excluding</u> the charge for anesthesia time?

61. During the last month, did you administer anesthesia for an appendectomy?*

    a. How many of these operations did you administer anesthesia for during the last month?

    b. How many units are included in the base charge for that procedure, assuming no unusual complications and <u>excluding</u> the charge for anesthesia time?

62. During the last month, did you administer anesthesia for a cholecystectomy?*

    a. How many of these operations did you administer anesthesia for during the last month?

    b. How many units are included in the base charge for that procedure, assuming no unusual complications and <u>excluding</u> the charge for anesthesia time?

<u>Pathology</u>

63. What is your current usual fee for...

    a. a consulation during surgery including frozen section?

    b. a pathological examination of a surgical specimen, gross and microscopic?

    c. an autopsy, gross and microscopic examination?

64. During the last week, did you personally interpret or direct technicians who interpreted clinical chemistry tests that were done on automated multichannel equipment?

    a. How many of these clinical chemistry or chemistry tests did you interpret or were interpreted under your supervision during the last week?

    b. Including lab fees, what is the current usual charge for a chemistry test?

65. During the last week, did you personally interpret or direct technicians who interpreted a complete blood count?*

    a. How many of these procedures were interpreted by you or were interpreted under your direction during that week?

    b. Including lab fees, what is the current usual charge for that procedure?

---

*Parts a and b of the question are asked only if the response is "yes".

-133-

66. During the last week, did you personally interpret or direct technicians who interpreted a routine, complete urinanalysis?*
   a. How many of these procedures were interpreted by you or were interpreted under your direction during that week?
   b. Including lab fees, what is the current usual charge for that procedure?

67. During the last week, did you personally interpret or direct technicians who interpreted cervical pap smears?*
   a. How many of these procedures were interpreted by you or were interpreted under your direction during that week?
   b. Including lab fees, what is the current usual charge for that procedure?

68. During the last week, did you personally interpret or direct technicians who interpreted body fluid cytopathology?*
   a. How many of these procedures were interpreted by you or were interpreted under your direction during that week?
   b. Including lab fees, what is the current usual charge for that procedure?

HOSPITAL UTILIZATION**

All specialties except radiology, anesthesiology and pathology

69. In your last complete week of practice, how many patients did you personally discharge from the hospital?

70. Among those patients that you discharged in that week, what has been the average length of stay in days in the hospital?

QUARTERLY INCOME AND EXPENSES

71. Whether or not your practice is incorporated, are you a full or part-owner of your main medical practice?***   (IF YES, GO TO Q. 72)
   a. Are you an employee of a hospital?***   (IF YES, GO TO Q. 75)

72. Is your main practice organized as a solo practice, a partnership, group practice, or some other type of association?

Solo, self-employed physicians Only

73. In the [last calendar quarter] what were your total tax-deductible professional expenses from medical practice to the nearest $1,000?

---

*Parts a and b of the question are asked only if the response is "yes".
**Hospital utilization questions were first asked in the 3rd quarter 1982 survey.
***In the 1st through 3rd quarter 1982 surveys the following question was used in place of Q.71 as it appears above: "In your main medical practice, are you self-employed or employed by a private practice, hospital or other medical facility?"

74. In the [last calendar quarter], what was your share of your practice's total tax-deductible professional expenses to the nearest $1,000?
    a. Did you have any other tax-deductible professional expenses during this period that were not included in the amount you just gave?*
    b. What were these other professional expenses to the nearest $1,000?

All physicians

75. During the [last calendar quarter], what was your own income from medical practice to the nearest $1,000 after expenses but before taxes? Please include all income from fees, salaries, retainers, fringe benefits and other forms of compensation.

76. Were any contributions made into pension, profit sharing or other deferred compensation plans for you during the last calendar quarter]?*
    a. How much was contributed for you for the period to the nearest $1,000?
    b. Did you include (this amount/deferred compensation) in the income figure you gave?

77. During the [last calendar quarter], did you miss any weeks of practice because of illness, vacation or for any other reason?*
    a. How many weeks did you not practice during this period?

===

CORE AND SPECIAL TOPICS QUESTIONS

===

PHYSICIAN FINANCIAL CONTRACTS WITH HOSPITALS
(4th Quarter 1981 Survey)

78. Do you have a financial contract or agreement, oral or written, with any hospital for your services?   [IF "NO", SKIP Q. 79-81]

79. Hospitals arrange various types of compensation with physicians. Under your arrangement, do you receive any part of your compensation from...
    a. a salary?
    b. a percentage of gross department billings?
    c. a percentage of net department revenues?
    d. a fee-for-service or from a fixed percentage of each charge?
    e. a minimum guaranteed income combined with another form of compensation?
    f. some other method of compensation?

80. Did your arrangement with the hospital include a lease agreement?

---

*Remaining parts of the question are not asked if the response is "no".

81. What percentage of your own net income during the third quarter of 1981 was derived from financial contracts or agreements with hospitals?

AMBULATORY SURGERY
(1st Quarter 1982 Survey)

All specialties except psychiatry, radiology, anesthesiology and pathology

82. During the last month, did you perform any operations or assists, either on an ambulatory or inpatient basis?   [IF "NO", GO TO Q. 83]
    a. About how many operations and assists did you perform altogether during the past month both on an ambulatory and inpatient basis?
    b. Were any of these operations or assists performed on an ambulatory basis?   [IF "NO", GO TO Q. 83]
    c. What percent of the operations and assists that you performed last month were on an ambulatory basis?
    d. Do you use any of the following settings to perform ambulatory surgery?
       -- hospital ambulatory surgery center
       -- free-standing ambulatory surgery center
       -- your office
       -- some other location
    e. Which of the settings [just mentioned] do you use most often to perform ambulatory surgery?

83. Thinking back to two years ago, did you perform any operations or assists on an ambulatory basis at that time?
                                        [IF "NO", DO NOT ASK PART A]
    a. Would you say that you currently perform a greater percent , about the same percent or a lesser percent of your operations and assists on an ambulatory basis than two years ago?

MEDICAL TECHNOLOGY DIFFUSION
(1st Quarter 1982 Survey)

84. During the last 12 months, did you use any of the following sources of information to learn about new diagnostic and therapeutic procedures?
    a. Medical journals.
    b. Professional meetings, conferences or continuing education courses.
    c. Discussions with other physicians.
    d. Technological assessments produced by government agencies.
    e. Any other sources.

88. How would you rank the sources you mentioned in terms of their importance in learning about new diagnostic and therapeutic procedures?
    a. Medical journals
    b. Professional meetings, conferences or continuing education courses.

c. Discussions with other physicians.
d. Technological assessments produced by government agencies.
e. Other sources.

89. During the past twelve months, did you perform for the first time any new diagnostic or therapeutic procedure that reflected advances in medical knowledge or technology?　　　　[IF "NO", GO TO Q. 90]
    a. During this period, how many different dianostic or therapeutic procedures did you perform for the first time?

92. During the past twelve months, did you drop any procedures from your normal office routine as a result of changes in medical knowledge or technology?　　　　　　[IF "NO", GO TO Q.91]
    a. How many procedures did you drop because of changes in medical knowledge and technology?
    b. How many of these procedures that you dropped were replaced by new procedures?

91. During the past 12 months, did you learn about any new diagnostic or therapeutic procedures that were relevant to your practice, but which you chose not to adopt in your practice activities?
    　　　　　　　　　　　　　　　　　　　　[IF "NO", SKIP PART A]
    a. Please [indicate] whether your decision not to adopt new procedures was based on any of these reasons:
       1. There was insufficient information about the medical safety and effectiveness of the procedure.
       2. You do not have necessary equipment or facilities.
       3. The procedure is currently performed at a hospital or other facility in the area.
       4. The cost of the procedure was too great relative to the expected patient benefits.

1982 CORE SURVEY QUESTIONS:
1981 INCOME AND EXPENSES AND WAITING TIME
(2nd Quarter 1982 Survey)

<u>Self-employed physicians only</u>

92. In 1981, what (were your/was your share of your practice's) total tax-deductible professional expenses from medical practice to the nearest $1,000?*

93. In 1981, what (were your/was your share of your practice's) total tax-deductible professional expenses for the following items to the nearest $1,000?*
    a. Total nonphysician payroll expenses including fringe benefits.
    b. Professional medical liability insurance premiums.
    c. Depreciation, leases and rent on medical equipment.
    d. Office expenses, including rent, mortgage, utilities and telephone.

---

*First wording in parentheses is used for physicians in solo practice; second wording is used for physicians in non-solo practice.

e. Medical materials and supplies, such as drugs, x-ray films and expenses for outside lab work, drugs and other services.

All physicians

94. During 1981, what was your own net income from medical practice to the nearest $1,000 after expenses, but before taxes? Please include all income from fees, salaries, retainers, fringe benefits and other forms of compensation.

95. Were any contributions made into pension, profit-sharing or deferred compensation plans for you during 1981?

    [IF "NO", GO TO Q.96]

    a. How much was contributed for you to the nearest $1,000?
    b. Did you include this amount in the income figure you gave me?

96. How many weeks did you practice in 1981? Please do not include vacations, illness, medical meetings, military service or other similar absences from practice.

All specialties except radiology, anesthesiology and pathology

97. How many days does a new patient wishing to see you typically have to wait for an appointment?

98. How many minutes does a patient typically have to wait to see you after arriving for a scheduled appointment?

NON-PHYSICIAN PERSONNEL
(2nd Quarter 1982 Survey)

Non-physician personnel

99. The next set of questions relate to personnel in your practice and under your immediate supervision. How many positions do you have for the following type of personnel on a full-time equivalent basis, whether currently filled or not?
    a. Registered nurses
    b. Licensed practical nurses
    c. Nurse practitioners
    d. Physicians assistant
    e. Secretaries, receptionists, and clerks
    f. X-ray technicians
    g. Medical laboratory technicians
    h. Respiratory therapists and technicians
    i. Physician therapists
    j. Radiation therapists
    k. EEG technologists
    l. Occupational therapists
    m. Perfusionists
    n. Medical assistants

100. How many physicians, if any, share the time of [type of personnel] in your practice with you?*

101. Are all of the positions that you have for [type of personnel] currently filled?*

102. How many vacancies do you currently have on a full-time equivalent basis for [type of personnel]?**

MALPRACTICE CLAIMS EXPERIENCE
(2nd Quarter 1982 Survey)

103. How many malpractice claims have been filed against you in your medical career?   [IF "NONE", SKIP Q.104-105]

104. How many of these claims were filed in the last 5 years?
                                                      [IF "NONE", SKIP Q.105]

105. Of the claims filed against you in the last 5 years, how many have had the following outcomes?
    a. Dismissal of suit.
    b. Settlement out-of-court.
    c. Acquitted in court trial.
    d. Conviction in court trial.

PHYSICIAN/HOSPITAL RELATIONS
(3rd Quarter 1982 Survey)

106. At how many different hospitals, if any, do you have admitting privileges?

107. The next several questions [Q.108-115] relate to the hospital at which you admit most of your patients. Is that hospital government non-federal, government federal, church operated non-profit, other non-profit, or for-profit investor-owned?

108. How many beds does the hospital at which you admit most of your patients have?

109. Does that hospital have a full-time hospital-employed medical director?   [IF "NO", GO TO Q.110]
    a. Does the medical director represent the interests of the medical staff?
    b. Does the medical director strengthen physician-hospital relationships?
    c. Does the medical director provide effective medical staff organizational services?

---

*Question is asked for each of the types of personnel which the response to Question 99 is greater than zero.
**Question is asked for each of the types of personnel for which the response to Question 101 is "no".

110. Are medical staff physicians represented on the governing board of the hospital?   [IF "NO", GO TO Q.111]
a. Do those physicians adequately represent the interests of the medical staff?

111. Are hospital long-range planning issues that significantly affect patient care and clinical services brought before the medical staff for review and consideration?

112. Are you concerned about competition from that hospital for patients and medical services?

113. Does that hospital presently have a sufficient number of physicians on its medical staff?

114. Are any departments of clinical services in that hospital not open to appointments of new, qualified medical practitioners?

115. Is that hospital part of a multihospital system?

PHYSICIAN RESPONSES TO COMPETITION
(4th Quarter 1982 Survey)

All specialties except radiology, anesthesiology and pathology

116. In the last month, how many housecalls, if any, did you make?

117. Thinking back to two years ago, how many housecalls, if any, did you make in a typical month?

118. How many hours, if any, do you currently schedule for evening or weekend office visits in a typical week?

119. Thinking back to two years ago, how many hours did you schedule for evening or weekend office visits in a typical week?

All specialties

120. Currently, how many full-time equivalent non-physician employees are under your supervision?

121. Two years ago, how many full-time equivalent non-physician employees were under your supervision?

Self-employed physicians only

122. Within the last five years, which of the following have you done?
a. Located your practice in a non-traditional setting such as a shopping center or store front.
b. Opened a satellite office or ambulatory care center, either alone or with other physicians.
c. Used surveys to learn about patient satisfaction with various aspects of your practice.

d. Developed a patient newsletter.
e. Studied demographic information on your community for its effects on your practice in coming years.
f. Advertised your practice on radio or TV or in a newspaper or magazine.
g. Employed an advertising, public relations or marketing firm or consultant.
h. Developed a written marketing plan for your practice.

123. Are you considering participating in a program to learn more about marketing concepts and techniques within the next two years?

IMPACT OF THE ECONOMY ON PHYSICIANS
(4th Quarter 1982 Survey)

All specialties except radiology, anesthesiology, and pathology

124. What percent of your patient visits in the last month were with patients who have become unemployed and lost their health insurance coverage in the last year?

125. What percent of your patient visits in the last month were with patients who have lost their Medicaid coverage due to program cut-backs in the last year?

Fee-for-service physicians only

126. Are you currently providing any free or reduced fee care to patients who have become unemployed and lost their health insurance coverage in the last year?   [IF "NO", GO TO Q.127]
a. By what percent has this reduced your billings in the last month?

127. Are you currently providing any free or reduced fee care to patients who have lost their Medicaid coverage in the last year due to program cutbacks?   [IF "NO", GO TO Q.128]
a. By what percent has this reduced your billings in the last month?

128. Are you currently participating in an organized fair share program -- that is, a health care program for community wide response to problems of the unemployed and needy?

1983 CORE SURVEY QUESTIONS:
TYPE OF PRACTICE, 1981 INCOME AND EXPENSES AND WAITING TIME
(2nd Quarter 1983 Survey)

129. Whether or not your practice is incorporated, are you a full or part owner of your main medical practice?   [IF "YES", GO TO Q.130]
a. In your main practice, are you employed by a hospital?
[IF "YES", GO TO 132]
b. In your main practice, are you employed either by a government agency or by a facility owned and operated by a government agency?   [IF "YES", GO TO 132]

130. Which of the following legal forms of organization best describes your main practice: sole proprietorship, partnership professional corporation, investor-owned for profit corporation, or some other form of organization?

131. Including yourself, how many physicians are in your main practice?

132. In what year did you begin medical practice after completing your undergraduate and graduate medical training?

Self-employed physicians only

133. For each of [the following] expense items, what (were your/was your share of your practice)* tax-deductible professional expenses in 1982 to the nearest $1,000? (If you had any other professional expenses that were not related to your main practice, include these expenses as well.)**
    a. Total non-physician payroll expenses, including fringe benefits.
    b. Professional medical liability, or malpractice, insurance premiums.
    c. Depreciation, leases and rent on medical equipment.
    d. Office expenses, including rent, mortgage, utilities and telephone.
    e. Medical materials and supplies, such as drugs, x-ray films and expenses for outside lab work and other services.
    f. Professional car upkeep and depreciation.
    g. Professional association memberships, professional journals and continuing education.
    h. Other medical expenses that [have not been mentioned], any contributions for you into deferred compensation plans.

134. Altogether then, your (share of your practice's)** tax-deductible expenses from medical practice in 1982 were [TOTAL EXPENSES]. Is that correct?***

---

  * First wording is used for physicians in solo practice; second wording is used for physicians in non-solo practice.

 ** Wording in parentheses is used only for physicians in non-solo practices.

*** TOTAL EXPENSES is computed as the sum of the responses to individual parts of Q.133. If the physician answers "no" to Q.134, then Q.133 is repeated. If the physician refused to respond or responded "don't know" to any part of Q.133, then the following question(s) were used as a substitute for Q.134.

   S134. In 1982 what (were your/was your share of your practice's)* total tax-deductible professional expenses from medical practice to the nearest $1,000? Do not include contributions that were made for you into deferred compensation plans.

   S134A. Physicians in non-solo practice only: Did you have any other tax-deductible professional expenses during 1982 that were not included in the amount you just gave me?

             [IF "NO", SKIP PART A]

      a. What were these other professional expenses to the nearest $1,000?

<u>All physicians</u>

135. During 1982, what was your own net income from medical practice to the nearest $1,000? Please include all incomes from fees, salaries retainers and other forms of compensation.

136. Were any contributions made for you into pension, profit-sharing or other deferred compensation plans during 1982?

[IF "NO", GO TO Q.137]

a. How much was contributed for you during 1982 to the nearest $1,000?

b. Did you include this amount in the income figure you just gave me?

<u>Physicians in non-solo practice only</u>

137. Which of the following methods of income compensation is your main source of income from medical practice: fee-for-service, salary, percent of net billings or profit, percent of gross billings, or some other method?

<u>All physicians</u>

138. How many weeks did you practice in 1982? Please do not include vacations, sick times, ambulatory service or other similar absences from practice.

<u>All specialties except radiology, anesthesiology and pathology</u>

139. How many days does a new patient wishing to see you typically have to wait for an appointment?

140. How many minutes does a patient typically have to wait to see you after arriving for a scheduled appointment?

Appendix B

DEFINITIONS AND COMPUTATION PROCEDURES

This appendix describes definitions and computation procedures used in reporting information from the AMA Socioeconomic Monitoring System (SMS). Changes in methodology over time relating to specific types of information for which trends are reported in the detailed tabulations in Socioeconomic Characteristics of Medical Practice (the "Gray Book") are also discussed. Most of these changes in methodology relate to differences between SMS surveys and the AMA Periodic Surveys of Physicians (PSPs) on which data for years prior to 1981 is based. These changes should be carefully noted in making comparisons of data for years prior to and since 1981.

Questions from SMS surveys referenced in this appendix are found in Appendix A. Tables referred to are those contained in the Gray Book detailed tabulations.

Sample Population

The population from which samples are drawn for SMS surveys includes all active non-federal office-based and hospital-based physicians as defined by the AMA Physician Masterfile.* The population from which samples were drawn for the PSPs differed by the exclusion of hospital-based physicians. This difference should be recognized in any comparison between data in the PSPs and SMS surveys.

Specialty

Specialty classifications used in reporting SMS data are shown in Figure 1. Specialty is determined from responses to Question 1 in SMS surveys. The question used in PSPs from 1973 through 1980 to determine specialty was as follows: "Please give the specialty from which you derived 50% or more of your medical income in [the last year]."

Census Region and Division

States included in each Census region and division are shown in Figure 2. The state in which each physician was located is identified from the AMA Physician Masterfile.

---

*Classifications used in the AMA Physician Masterfile are defined in M. Eiler, Physician Characteristics and Distribution, 1982 Edition (American Medical Association, 1983).

FIGURE 1

SMS Survey Specialty Classifications

SMS SPECIALTY CLASSIFICATION	AMA PHYSICIAN MASTERFILE SPEICALTIES
General/Family Practice	
General/Family Practice	General Practice, Family Practice
Medical Specialties	
Internal Medicine	Allergy, Cardiovascular Diseases, Gastroenterology, Internal Medicine, Pulmonary Diseases
Pediatrics:	General Surgery, Neurosurgery, Ophthalmology, Orthopedic Surgery, Plastic Surgery, Colon and Rectal Surgery, Thoracic Surgery, Urology
Surgical Specialties	
Surgery:	Pediatrics, Pediatric Allergy, Pediatric Cardiology
Obstetrics/Gynecology:	Obstetrics and Gynecology
Other Specialties	
Radiology:	Radiology, Diagnostic Radiology, Therapeutic Radiology
Psychiatry:	Psychiatry, Child Psychiatry
Anesthesiology:	Anesthesiology
Pathology:	Forensic Pathology, Pathology
Other:	Aerospace Medicine, Neurology, Occupational Medicine, Physical Medicine and Rehabilitation, General Preventive Medicine, Public Health, Dermatology, Emergency Medicine, Other Specialty, Unspecified.

FIGURE 2

Census Region and Division Definitions

CENSUS REGION AND DIVISION	STATES

Northeast

New England: Connecticut, Maine, Massachusetts, New Hampshire, Rhode Island, Vermont

Middle Atlantic: New Jersey, New York, Pennsylvania

North Central

East North Central: Illinois, Indiana, Michigan, Ohio, Wisconsin

West North Central: Iowa, Kansas, Minnesota, Missouri, Nebraska, North Dakota, South Dakota

South

South Atlantic: Delaware, District of Columbia, Florida, Georgia, Maryland, North Carolina, South Carolina, Virginia, West Virginia

East South Central: Alabama, Kentucky, Mississippi, Tennessee

West South Central: Arkansas, Louisiana, Oklahoma, Texas

West

Mountain: Arizona, Colorado, Idaho, Montana, Nevada, New Mexico, Utah, Wyoming

Pacific: Alaska, California, Hawaii, Oregon, Washington

Type of Practice

Physicians in solo and non-solo practices were distinguished in 1982 SMS surveys on the basis of responses to Question 72. Type of practice (solo vs. non-solo) was determined in the 1983 SMS core survey from responses to Question 131. Questions similar to either Question 72 or 131 in the SMS surveys were included in each of the PSPs.

Location

The location classification groups physicians into nonmetropolitan areas, metropolitan areas with a population less than one million persons and metropolitan areas with a population of one million or more persons. This classification was made on the basis of the demographic county classification contained on the AMA Physician Masterfile.

Employment Status

Employment status is determined for 1982 SMS surveys from responses to Question 71. The change in the wording of this question made in the 4th quarter of 1982 reflected the observation made while monitoring telephone interviews that some physicians (who were whole or part owners of an incorporated practice) were identifying themselves as employees. Employment status was determined in the 1983 SMS core survey on the basis of responses to Question 129. The PSPs provided no basis from which to ascertain employment status.

Age

The age of each physician in PSP and SMS surveys was determined from birthdate information on the AMA Physician Masterfile.

Weeks Practiced per Year (Table 1 and 2)

Data on weeks practiced in 1981 and 1982 is based on responses to Questions 96 and 138 respectively in the SMS surveys. Similar questions in the PSPs provided information on weeks practiced for years prior to 1981.

Hours in Professional Activities per Week (Table 3)

Professional activities includes all patient care activities, administrative activities connected with medical practice and other professional activities that do not involve patient care such as medical staff functions, teaching and research. Hours per week in professional activities in 1982 is based on "TOTAL HOURS" as calculated for purposes of Question 5, 8, 11, 14, or 17 (depending on physician specialty) in the SMS surveys.

Hours in Patient Care Activities per Week (Tables 4 and 5)

Patient care activities include direct patient care and activities related to patient care, such as interpreting lab tests and x-rays and consulting with other physicians. Hours per week in patient care activities in 1982 is based on the sum of the responses to parts a-g of Question 4, parts a-d of Question 7, parts a-e of Question 10, parts a-f of Question 13, or parts a-e of Question 16 (depending on physician specialty) in the SMS surveys. Hours per week in patient care activities for 1973 through 1980 was determined from responses to the second of the following questions included in the PSPs:

1. How many total hours did you practice during your most recent complete week of practice (exclude "on call" hours not actually worked)?

2. How many of these hours were spent in providing DIRECT patient care or patient related services (include patients' lab tests, interpreting x-rays, etc; exclude administrative tasks, meetings, etc.)?

Hours in patient care activities for 1973 through 1980, as defined here, was previously termed hours in direct patient care in the Profile of Medical Practice series published by the AMA.

Hours in Direct Patient Care Activities per Week (Table 6)

Direct patient care activities include seeing patients in the office, on hospital rounds, in surgery and in other settings. Hours per week in direct patient care activities in 1982 was determined for all specialties except psychiatry, radiology, anesthesiology and pathology from SMS surveys from the sum of reponses to parts a-f of Question 4. Since a different classification of patient care activities was asked about in SMS surveys among physicians in psychiatry, radiology, anesthesiology, and pathology (as reflected by Questions 7-18), physicians in these specialties are not reflected in computations of direct patient care hours in Table 6 is based.

Office Hours and Hours on Hospital Rounds per Week (Tables 7-10)

Office hours and hours on hospital rounds per week in 1982 are based on responses to Questions 4a and 4c respectively in the SMS surveys. Physicians in psychiatry, radiology, anesthesiology and pathology were not asked Questions 4a and 4c and are, therefore, not reflected in the data on office hours and hours in hospital rounds in 1982 reported in Tables 7-10. Data on office hours and hours on hospital rounds for years prior to 1982 included in Tables 8 and 10 are based on PSP surveys. The questions used to collect this information in the PSPs were similar to those in the SMS surveys. Although questions on office hours and hours on hospital rounds were asked of physicians in all specialties in the PSPs, responses from physicians in psychiatry, radiology, anesthesiology, and pathology were excluded in computations made for Tables 8 and 10 to make data for years prior to 1982 comparable to the data for 1982 from the SMS surveys. The specialty exclusions account for differences in data for years prior to 1982 in Tables 8 and 10, other than for individual specialties, from data previously reported in the Profile of Medical Practice series.

Hours in Surgery per Week (Table 11)

Hours in surgery per week in 1982 is based on responses to Question 4b in the SMS surveys. Physicians in psychiatry, radiology, anesthesiology and pathology were not asked Question 4b and are, therefore, not reflected in the data on hours in surgery per week reported in Table 11.

Total Patient Visits per Week (Tables 12 and 13)

Total patient visits includes visits in the office, on hospital rounds, in hospital emergency rooms and outpatient clinics and in all other settings. Total patient visits per week in 1982 is based on the sum of responses to parts a, c, d, e and f of Question 6 in the SMS surveys. Physicians in psychiatry, radiology, anesthesiology, and pathology were not asked Question 6 and are, therefore, not reflected in the data for 1982 in Tables 12 and 13. Questions from the PSPs on which data on total patient visits per week for years 1975 through 1980 are as follows:

1975

Please indicate the number of patient visits in the following categories for your most recent complete week of practice:
a. Office
b. Hospital (inpatient only)
c. Nursing home
d. Emergency room
e. Other

1976, 1978, 1979

How many patient visits did you have during your most recent complete week of practice. . .
a. at the office?
b. at the hospital?
c. at all other services (or facilities)?

1980

How many total patient visits did you have during your most complete week of practice (include all patient contacts other than telephone).

Although questions on visits were asked of physicians in all specialties in the PSPs, responses from physicians in psychiatry, radiology, anesthesiology and pathology were excluded in computations made for Table 13 to make data for 1975 through 1980 comparable to the data for 1982 from the

SMS surveys. The specialty exclusions account for differences in data for years prior to 1982 in Table 13, other than for individual specialties, from data previously reported in the Profiles of Medical Practice series.

Office Visits and Visits on Hospital Rounds per Week (Tables 14-17)

Office visits and visits on hospital rounds per week in 1982 are based on responses to Questions 6a and 6c respectively in the SMS surveys. Physicians in psychiatry, radiology, anesthesiology and pathology were not asked Questions 6a and 6c and are, therefore, not reflected in the data in Tables 14-17. Data on office visits and visits on hospital rounds for years prior to 1982 included in Tables 15 and 17 are based on PSP surveys. The questions used to collect this information in the PSPs were similar to those in the SMS surveys. Although questions on office visits and visits on hospital rounds were asked of physicians in all specialties in the PSPs, responses from physicians in psychiatry, radiology, anesthesiology and pathology were excluded in computing Tables 15 and 17 to make data for years prior to 1982 comparable to the data for 1982 from the SMS surveys. The specialty exclusions account for differences in data for years prior to 1982 in Tables 15 and 17, other than for individual specialties, from data previously reported in the Profile of Medical Practice series.

Surgical Procedures per Week (Table 18)

Surgical procedures per week in 1982 is based on responses to Question 6b in the SMS surveys. Physicians in psychiatry, radiology, anesthesiology and pathology were not asked Question 6b and are, therefore, not reflected in the data on surgical procedures per week reported in Table 18.

Patient Care Activities: Psychiatry (Table 19)

Hours and the number of sessions with individual patients per week in 1982 are respectively based on the sum of responses to parts a and b of Question 7 and responses to Question 9a in the SMS surveys. Hours and the number of sessions with family and non-family groups per week in 1982 are respectively based on responses to Question 7c and the sum of responses to Questions 9c and 9d in the SMS surveys.

Patient Care Activities: Radiology (Table 20)

Data on patient care activities of radiologists in 1982 in the columns from left to right in Table 20 are respectively based on responses to Questions 10a, 12a, 10b, 12b, 10c, 12c, 10e and 12e in the SMS surveys.

Patient Care Activities: Anesthesiology (Table 21)

Hours spent personally anesthetizing patients and the number of patients personally anesthetized per week in 1982 are respectively based on responses to Questions 13a and 15a in the SMS surveys. Hours spent supervising nurse anesthetists per week in 1982 is based on responses to Question 13b in the SMS surveys. The number of patients anesthetized by nurse anesthetists supervised by each anesthesiologist supervision is based on responses to Question 15b in the SMS surveys. Hours and the number of pre-anesthesia and other inpatient visits per week in 1982 are respectively based on the sum of responses to Questions 13c and 13e and the sum of responses to Questions 15c and 15e respectively in the SMS surveys.

Patient Care Activities: Pathology (Table 23)

Data on patient care activities of pathologists in 1982 in the columns from left to right in Table 23 are respectively based on responses to Questions 16a, 18a, 16b, 18b, 16d, 18d, 16c, and 18c in the SMS surveys.

Waiting Time (Tables 24 and 25)

Data on waiting time to be scheduled for an appointment and waiting time in the physician's office after arriving for a scheduled appointment in 1982 are based on responses to Questions 97 and 98 respectively in the 1982 SMS core survey. Physicians in radiology, anesthesiology and pathology were not asked Questions 97 and 98 and are, therefore, not reflected in the data on waiting time in tables 24 and 25.

Hospital Utilization (Tables 25 and 26)

Data on patients discharged from the hospital per week and the length of stay of patients discharged in 1982 are based on responses to Question 69 and 70 in the SMS surveys. Physicians in radiology, anesthesiology and pathology were not asked Questions 69 and 70 and are, therefore, not reflected in the data on hospital utilization in Tables 25 and 26.

Fees Tables (27-32)

Fees for office visits with new patients, office visits with established patients and follow-up hospital visits in 1982 were obtained in SMS surveys from responses to Questions 20a, 20b, and 20c respectively or from responses to Questions 22a, 22b, and 22c respectively depending on physician specialty. In computing means and their standard errors for fees for each type of visit for 1982, the fee reported by each physician is weighted by the frequency with which the physician has that type of visit.* The frequency of new patient office visits is determined from re-

---

*Formulas for these means and standard errors are given in the section on computation procedures later in this appendix.

-152-

sponses to Question 6a1 in the SMS surveys. The frequency of office visits with established patients used in weighting fees for this type of visit is based on the response to Question 6a less the response to Question 6a1 and, if applicable for the specialty less the number of periodic or annual type exams per week based on the response to Question 26a or 27a divided by 3.9 (3.9, the average number of weeks practiced per month in 1982 based on responses to Question 138 in the 1983 core survey, is used to convert the monthly data on the number of periodic exams to a weekly basis). The frequency of hospital visits used in weighting fees for these visits is designed to exclude hospital visits included in fees for surgical or obstetrical procedures. Thus, the weight is based on responses to Question 6c less the number of hospital visits for which the fee is included in fees for surgical or obstetrical procedures as implied by responses to Questions 21 and 23. Physicians in psychiatry, radiology, anesthesiology and pathology were not asked questions on fees for the types of visits reflected in Tables 27-32 in the 1982 SMS surveys and are, therefore, not reflected in the 1982 data in those tables.

Data on fees for years prior to 1982 in Tables 28, 30 and 32 is based only on the following questions from the PSPs:

For each of the following procedures, indicate the number of times you perform the procedure during a typical complete week of practice and the current usual fee you charge for the procedure.

a. Office visit, new patient, brief evaluation, history, examination and/or treatment.

b. Office visit, established patient, brief examination, evaluation and/or treatment, same or new illness.

c. Hospital visit, new or established patient brief examination, evaluation and/or treatment, same illness.

Although these questions were asked of physicians in all specialties in the PSPs, responses from physicians in psychiatry, radiology, anesthesiology and pathology were excluded from the computations made for Tables 28, 30 and 32 to make data for years prior to 1982 comparable to data for 1982 from the SMS surveys. The specialty exclusions account for differences in data for years prior to 1982 in Tables 28, 30 and 32, other than for individual specialties, from data previously reported in the Profiles of Medical Practice series.*

Professional Expenses (Table 33-37)

Professional expense information reported in Tables 33-37 refers to tax-deductible professional expenses from medical practice. Data on total professional expenses for 1982 is based on "TOTAL EXPENSES" as calculated for purposes of Question 134 or on the response to Question S134 (plus

---

*No weights were used in computing means and their standard errors for fees for years prior to 1982 since the data necessary was not available from the PSPs for this purpose.

the response to Question S134A if that question was asked) in the 1983 SMS core survey. Data on individual expense components for 1982 in Table 37 is based on response to parts a-e of Question 133 from the 1983 SMS core survey. Data on professional expenses for 1981 in Tables 34 and 36 are based on responses to Question 92 from the 1982 SMS core survey. The change in the question used to obtain professional expense information between the 1982 and 1983 core surveys was designed to achieve a better reconciliation between total expenses and the amounts reported for individual expense components and to probe for professional expenses of physicians in non-solo practices that are not related to their main practice which might otherwise be missed. Data on professional expenses for years prior to 1981 reported in Tables 34 and 36 are based on responses to the following questions from the PSPs:

1973-75, 1977

What were your total professional expenses in [YEAR] to the nearest $1,000? (Include only those expenses that are allowable business deductions for Federal income tax purposes. If in practice with other physicians, give only your share of the practice's expenses.)

1978-1979

What were your total tax-deductible professional expenses in [YEAR]? (If you shared expenses with other physicians, indicate your share only.)

While data relating to professional expenses for 1981 and 1982 from the SMS surveys are based on only self-employed physicians, professional expense information for years prior to 1981 was obtained from all physicians responding to the PSPs. Note, however, that hospital-based physicians were not included in PSP samples.

Net Income (Tables 38-41)

Net income from medical practice is defined to include all earnings from medical practice after expenses but before taxes, including fringe benefits and contributions made into deferred compensation plans. Net income in 1982 was determined in the 1983 SMS core survey from responses to Question 135. In addition, Question 136 was included as a probe to ensure that deferred compensation plan contributions were fully represented in net income. If the physician responded "no" to Question 136b, the response given to Question 136a was added to the response to Question 135 to obtain net income. Question 94 and 95 in the 1982 SMS core survey were similarly used to obtain information on net income for 1981. The questions used in PSPs used to obtain net income information for years prior to 1981 included in Tables 39 and 41 were as follows:

1973

What was your individual net medical practice income before taxes in 1973 to the nearest $1,000 (your 1973 gross income minus your tax-deductible profesional expenses)?

What was your [YEAR] individual before tax net income from medical practice to the nearest \$1,000?

1979

What was your 1979 individual net income before taxes from medical practice? (Include all income from fees, salaries, retainers, etc., as well as the value of all fringe benefits paid on your behalf, e.g., Keogh Plan.)

Computation Procedures

Means (or averages) for all characteristics, except for 1982 fees, reported in the Gray Book and SMS Reports are estimated by simple averages of responses to the relevant questions in the PSPs and SMS surveys. Thus, if x_i represents the response from physician i concerning a particular characteristic and n physicians responded to the relevant survey question, the estimated mean of the characteristic and its standard error are given as follows:

(1) Mean:
$$\bar{x} = \frac{1}{n} \Sigma x_i$$

(2) Standard error:
$$\hat{\sigma}_{\bar{x}} = \left[\frac{\Sigma (x_i - \bar{x})^2}{n(n-1)} \right]^{1/2}$$

where Σ indicates the sumation over all n physicians.

Means for fees in 1982 are computed as weighted averages of fees reported by physicians in SMS surveys with the weight for each physician given by the frequency with which the physician performs the procedure. Thus, if x_i is the fee reported by physician i for a given procedure, w_i is the frequency with which physician i performs the procedure and n physicians provide information on the fee and frequency of performing the procedure, the estimated mean fee for the procedure and its standard error are given by:

(3) Mean:
$$\bar{x} = \frac{\Sigma w_i x_i}{\Sigma w_i}$$

(4) Standard error:
$$\hat{\sigma}_{\bar{x}} = \left[\frac{\Sigma w_i (x_i - \bar{x})^2}{n \Sigma w_i} \right]^{1/2}$$

In some instances, data from more than one SMS survey are combined for estimating the mean of a characteristic. This procedure was used for 1982 data on all characteristics except waiting time, professional expenses and net income included in the detailed tabulations in the Gray Book. In these cases, means are estimated with the same formulas as given above using the combined responses from the different surveys. However, since the samples for SMS surveys in each quarter include some physicians who were interviewed once before the previous quarter, the calculation of the standard errors must be modified to reflect the correlation of responses from physicians who have two responses included among the surveys that have been combined. The modified standard errors are given as:

$$\hat{\sigma}_{\bar{x}} \left(1 + 2\hat{\rho} \; \frac{n_r}{n} \right)^{1/2}$$

where $\hat{\sigma}_{\bar{x}}$ is given by either formula (2) or (4) above, depending on the characteristic, n is the total number of responses used in estimating the mean of the characteristic and $\hat{\sigma}_{\bar{x}}$ from the combined surveys, n_r is the number of physicians represented in the combined survey sample who provided information on the characteristic in two consecutive surveys and $\hat{\rho}$ is the estimated correlation coefficient of responses from physicians providing information on the characteristic in two consecutive surveys.